Practical Obs
Fistula Surg

CW01678385

To Dr Catherine Hamlin and the staff of the Addis Ababa Fistula Hospital – especially to Mamitu Gashe, the patient turned surgeon

Practical Obstetric Fistula Surgery

Brian Hancock MD FRCS
Honorary Consultant Surgeon,
University Hospital of South Manchester, Manchester, UK

Contributing Author
Andrew Browning MB BS MRCOG
Director, Bahr Dar Fistula Centre, Ethiopia

The ROYAL
SOCIETY of
MEDICINE
PRESS Limited

© 2009 Royal Society of Medicine Press Ltd

Published by the Royal Society of Medicine Press Ltd
1 Wimpole Street, London W1G 0AE, UK
Tel: +44 (0)20 7290 2921
Fax: +44 (0)20 7290 2929
Email: publishing@rsm.ac.uk
Website: www.rsmpress.co.uk

Apart from any fair dealing for the purposes of research or private study, criticism or review, as permitted under the UK Copyright, Designs and Patents Act, 1988, no part of this publication may be reproduced, stored or transmitted, in any form or by any means, without the prior permission in writing of the publishers or in the case of reprographic reproduction in accordance with the terms of licences issued by the Copyright Licensing Agency in the UK, or in accordance with the terms of licences issued by the appropriate Reproduction Rights Organization outside the UK. Enquiries concerning reproduction outside the terms stated here should be sent to the publishers at the UK address printed on this page.

The right of Brian Hancock to be identified as author of this work has been asserted by him in accordance with the Copyright, Designs and Patents Act, 1988.

British Library Cataloguing in Publication Data
A catalogue record for this book is available from the British Library

ISBN-13 978-1-85315-766-0

This publication is supported by educational grants from the Hamlin Churchill Childbirth Injuries Fund (UK charity no 257741; www.hamlinfistulauk.org) and the Uganda Childbirth Injuries Fund (UK charity no 10991354).

Distribution in Europe and Rest of World:

Marston Book Services Ltd
PO Box 269
Abingdon
Oxon OX14 4YN, UK
Tel: +44 (0)1235 465500
Fax: +44 (0)1235 465555
Email: direct.order@marston.co.uk

Distribution in the USA and Canada:

Royal Society of Medicine Press Ltd
c/o BookMasters, Inc
30 Amberwood Parkway
Ashland, Ohio 44805, USA
Tel: +1 800 247 6553 / +1 800 266 5564
Fax: +1 419 281 6883972 353 1303
Email: order@bookmasters.com

Distribution in Australia and New Zealand:

Elsevier Australia
30–52 Smidmore Street
Marrickville NSW 2204, Australia
Tel: +61 2 9517 8999
Fax: +61 2 9517 2249
Email: service@elsevier.com.au

Typeset by Phoenix Photosetting, Chatham, Kent
Printed and bound in Great Britain by Bell & Bain, Glasgow, UK

CONTENTS

Foreword

The term 'the developing world' suggests that all those living in it are moving forward in a positive way. Sadly, for millions of women this is just not the case. In spite of the United Nations fifth Millennium Development Goal of improving maternal health, there are no signs of any decrease in the number of women presenting with a vesico-vaginal fistula. This suggests that attempts at improving the situation, such as better education of women and availability of caesarean section, have been ineffective owing to lack of access to those at term or in early labour.

Fistula surgery has long been considered a specialist area. To a degree, it still is, but Brian Hancock's first book, *First Steps in Vesico-Vaginal Fistula Repair*, published in 2005, is now being used throughout the world to help train more surgeons and gynaecologists to repair fistulae, and in particular to aid them to identify those fistulae that beginners can safely repair and those that need to be referred to a specialist fistula surgeon.

This new book is one that should be read by anybody undertaking invasive procedures. The very clear lessons in it apply to us all.

It describes the extensive experience of two surgeons: Andrew Browning a gynaecologist and full-time fistula surgeon in Ethiopia, and Brian Hancock, a colorectal surgeon who has spent many months each year carrying out fistula repairs in Uganda and several countries in West Africa. They have both kept meticulous records of their experience and outcomes, and this book is about what they do and why they do it, supplemented at times with the experiences of a small number of other fistula surgeons.

The text is simple and clear. The authors quote another fistula surgeon, Kees Waaldijk – 'One surgeon in the vagina is already a crowd' – but despite this the photographs of the operative steps are superb.

The emphasis throughout is to avoid doing any more harm to these young women. There must be no misunderstanding as to which patients are suitable for the beginner and as to how they should be managed from the time of their presentation.

It is not just about closing the hole. The ischaemic insult that caused the fistula will have caused a series of other problems – social, psychiatric and physical – all of which require treatment. Even after closing the hole, the patient may still be wet as a result of severe stress incontinence. Andrew Browning's studies to identify those most at risk and of the use of a fibro-muscular sling are things of which all surgeons dealing with women with stress incontinence should be aware.

This book is an outstanding contribution to surgery in general and obstetric fistula surgery in particular, and should be studied and enjoyed by all those about to undertake or already undertaking this surgery.

Professor Gordon Williams MS FRCS FRCSEd FRCSGlas
Acting Medical Director and Urologist to the Addis Ababa Fistula Hospital
Dean, St Paul's Hospital Millennium Medical School, Addis Ababa, Ethiopia

Biographies

Brian Hancock MD FRCS is a retired colorectal surgeon from the University Hospital of South Manchester, UK. He first encountered obstetric fistulae while working as a general surgeon in Uganda 40 years ago, and performed simple repairs helped by Chassar Moir's classic textbook. He has made several visits to the Addis Ababa Fistula Hospital to learn and later to help with complex recto-vaginal fistulae. He is a trustee of Hamlin Fistula UK.

Since his retirement in 2000, he has spent 3 months a year in Africa, making visits to five hospitals in Uganda, and has worked as fistula surgeon and trainer with Mercy Ships in several West African countries.

Andrew Browning MB BS MRCOG is an Australian gynaecologist who for the last 6 years has been working in Ethiopia at the Addis Ababa Fistula Hospital (AAFH). He is now the director at the Bahr Dar Fistula Centre, a satellite of the AAFH in northern Ethiopia. He has trained surgeons from around the world, has several evidence-based publications and has been a speaker at a number of international meetings.

He regularly visits Uganda to help with training workshops at Kitovu Hospital with Brian Hancock and other surgeons.

Preface

The activities of the United Nations Population Fund 'End Fistula Campaign' and those of many other smaller organizations have done much to raise awareness of the vast scale of the problem of childbirth injury trauma in Africa and other poor countries. A declared objective is to train more surgeons and provide them with the right environment to practise.

My first book, *First Steps in Vesico-Vaginal Fistula Surgery*, has been popular with surgeons and nurses coming for training at the Addis Ababa Fistula Hospital, so I have been encouraged to produce a new book that will serve not only for the novice surgeon and team but also for those who are making progress up the long learning curve.

My own experience is limited to only a little over 1200 repairs, so I am very grateful to be able to collaborate with Dr Andrew Browning, a dedicated fistula surgeon on the staff of the Addis Ababa Fistula Hospital for the last 6 years. He now works at the satellite hospital in Bahr Dar, but has made many short-term visits to perform and teach fistula repairs at over ten different locations in six African countries. We have worked together on several occasions, and he is one of the most skilful surgeons I have seen, he is committed to personal audit and he already has several evidence-based publications on his results to his credit.

Fistula surgery does not belong to any one specialty. We believe that anyone with good surgical skills and knowledge of pelvic anatomy and an ability to adjust to the suboptimal conditions found in most poor countries can learn to repair the easier ones.

We strongly discourage specialists from developed countries from making one-off visits in the hope of contributing to the management of some 'challenging cases' or 'lending a hand'. The people most able to help fistula patients are those who work in Africa full time or make regular sustainable visits. It requires long-term commitment to learn the skills, as well as money to allow free treatment and to buy sutures, catheters and good instruments. Above all, it needs empathy and compassion for all that these patients have suffered.

It is a privilege to give a young woman a new start in life using basic surgical skills, and this has its own special rewards for the patient and the surgical team.

This publication has been sponsored by Hamlin Fistula UK (formerly Hamlin Churchill Childbirth Injuries Fund; UK Charity No. 257741; www.hamlinfistulauk.org) and by the Uganda Childbirth Injuries Fund (UK Charity No. 1099135).

INTRODUCTION

There is now a serious worldwide awareness of the vast number of untreated childbirth injury patients in Africa and other poor countries. The United Nations Population Fund 'End Fistula Campaign' and many other individual efforts are focusing on the prevention of fistulae through improved obstetric care. They also recognize the need to train more surgeons, especially nationals, but also overseas surgeons who are willing to provide resources and long-term commitment.

Nobody knows how many fistula patients there are who have been forgotten and are without hope. Estimates are up to two million in Africa alone. In Ethiopia, it is thought that there are 9000 new cases a year.

Fistula surgery has a justifiable reputation for being difficult, but it is not sufficiently appreciated that a significant number of cases are quite easy to cure.

Even experts cannot cure every case, however. The most experienced surgeons claim that 95% of fistulae can be closed (but they may have to operate on up to 10% a second or third time to achieve this figure). Closure of the fistula, however, does not always mean that the patient will be dry. Some 15–20% will have severe stress incontinence because the urethra and bladder have been so badly damaged. A few may improve in time, but, for those who do not, the operation has failed. Secondary operations for stress are possible, but have uncertain results. A reasonably experienced surgeon who takes on almost all the cases seen can at best probably only make 65–75% really dry.

Of course, the surgeon who turns down the difficult cases will have much better results. This explains the paradox that the better one is at repairing fistulae, the worse will be the results, because the expert rarely turns anyone away.

Anyone who watches a master fistula surgeon at work will marvel at the ease with which he or she demonstrates the art of fistula surgery. Even experienced surgeons who come new to fistula surgery will be surprised at how demanding the operations are and how difficult they seem at the start. The distorted anatomy and rigidity of tissues come as a shock. One not only has to know what must be done but also have the skill to do it. Accurate suturing in a confined space is difficult and requires more than average manual dexterity. There is a long learning curve owing to the complexity of many cases, and experience can only be gained by hands-on work. At present, the very few training opportunities are over-subscribed. The books available to help apprentice fistula surgeons are reviewed in Appendix A; these are at present either too complex for some or lacking in specific advice to provide all the help that a novice fistula surgeon requires.

There is no intention here to include a review of the literature, as this has recently been done very well,[1,2] nor can we cover every aspect of fistula surgery. We are limited by our own experience, which is constantly growing.

This book is above all intended as a user-friendly guide for those new to fistula surgery and those who are progressing up the long learning curve.

Our experiences are different in that Andrew Browning works as a full-time fistula surgeon in Ethiopia and Brian Hancock, who formerly worked as a general surgeon in Uganda, is a regular visiting surgeon to hospitals in East and West Africa.

Both of us have had the privilege of working in the well-provided environments of the Addis Ababa Fistula Hospital in Ethiopia and the Mercy Ships in West Africa. We have, however, both worked on a regular short-term basis in many mission or government hospitals that can provide only the basic facilities for fistula care. We therefore believe in a flexible approach that can be adapted to local circumstances where availability of materials and facilities varies widely. Our recommendations are largely directed to those working with restricted resources.

Teaching fistula surgery has been a large component of our work. It is rare for us to operate without at least one serious trainee present. Having helped many surgeons perform their first fistula operations, we can see the difficulties that they encounter and we understand the advice that they need. Some of our operations have been performed in hospitals that have had no prior experience of fistula surgery, and this is no bar to success.

While the text of this book is based on our own practical experience of what works best for us, we have been fortunate to visit or meet most of the small band of very experienced fistula surgeons in the world. We are most grateful for all that we have learnt from them, and many of their words of wisdom are incorporated in our advice.

There is little evidence-based research to guide a fistula surgeon, and many experts have evolved their own way of doing things in relative isolation. This is confusing for the trainee, and we cannot possibly give definitive advice, but we have tried to provide a balanced approach where possible.

There is no absolutely right way of repairing fistulae – there may be several routes to success, as long as general principles are followed.

It is important to appreciate that fistula surgery is constantly evolving as new evidence becomes available. Who would have predicted that the fat graft that for decades has been accepted as a vital component in fistula repair in the Addis Ababa Fistula Hospital would now be rarely used by many surgeons?

We expect that many of the views expressed in this book will be challenged and changed over time. Only the basic principles should stay the same. There is currently much more communication between fistula surgeons, and we expect to see considerable advances in our understanding and management of the complex issues in the near future.

The complexity of cases varies enormously: 25% are reasonably simple, 50% present a variety of technical challenges and the final 25% can be extremely challenging to cure.

Specialized centres are few and far between, and it is unrealistic to expect that fistulae should only be repaired at these centres. However, the complex cases should certainly be referred to established centres if possible.

We know of many instances where excellent work is being done in both independent and government hospitals by interested national, expatriate or regular visiting surgeons, provided that they recognize their limitations and do not attempt cases beyond their capability.

Nursing care is just as important as the surgery, and we show how care can be simplified and adapted to local circumstances. It is the surgeon's responsibility to be familiar with and to supervise all aspects of pre- and postoperative care.

We cannot over-emphasize that a fistula patient has more than just a hole in the bladder. The whole person is damaged by the disastrous outcome of obstructed labour. A full understanding of what the patient has suffered, her social background and her future are just as important to healing as the surgery.

In this book, we concentrate on the physical aspects of management, as no amount of empathy with the patient is of use unless they can be relieved of their constant incontinence as a first step. For an account of the holistic approach to the fistula patient, the reader is referred to the recent WHO manual described in Appendix A.

References

1. Wall LL, Arrowsmith SD, Briggs ND, Browning A, Lassey A. The obstetric vesico-vaginal fistula in the developing world. *Obstet Gynaecol Surv* 2005; **60**(suppl 1): S3–51.
2. Zheng AX, Anderson FWJ. Obstetric fistula in low-income countries. *Int J Gynecol Obstet* 2008; Nov 21 (Epub ahead of print).

1 Obstetric Fistulae: Cause and Nature; the Obstetric Fistula Complex; Classification

Understanding the cause and nature of vesico-vaginal fistulae

Obstetric vesico-vaginal fistulae (VVFs) are caused simply by unrelieved obstructed labour. Prolonged pressure of the baby's head against the back of the pubic bone produces ischaemic necrosis of the intervening soft tissues, i.e. some part of the genital tract and bladder (Figure 1.1). In a labour that is sufficiently prolonged to produce this, the baby almost always dies. The head then softens and the mother eventually delivers a stillborn infant (if she survives that long).

When the baby's head is stuck deep in the pelvis, the most common site for ischaemic injury is the urethro-vesical junction, but injury can also occur in other positions, either in isolation or together as one massive defect (Figure 1.2).

The extent of the injury depends on the duration of labour and the strength of the mother to survive this ordeal. In the most severe cases, ischaemia will affect the whole of the anterior wall of the vagina, the bladder base, much of the urethra and sometimes the rectum as well, leading to a recto-vaginal fistula. In the most extreme cases, the bladder is completely destroyed. Varying degrees of vaginal stenosis are

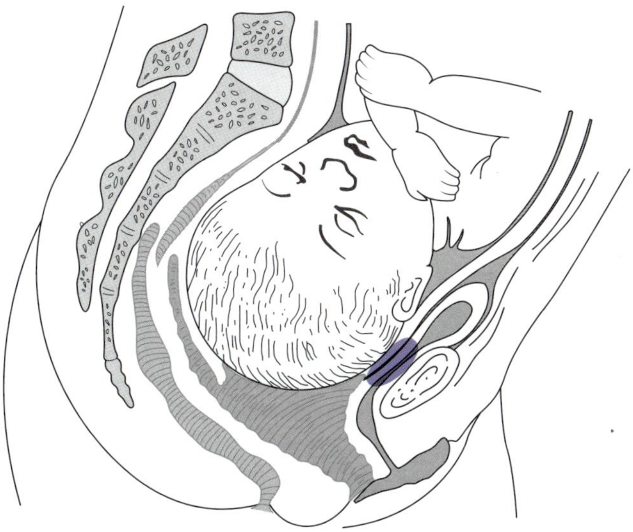

Figure 1.1 The area coloured blue is the first to undergo ischaemic necrosis.

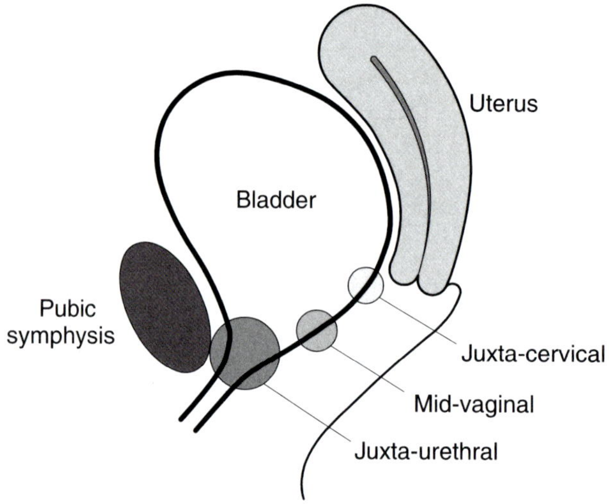

Figure 1.2 The various positions of ischaemic injury.

common. The exact site, size and amount of scar are functions of the position of the baby's head when it becomes stuck, and the duration of the obstruction.

Many mothers die of exhaustion or a ruptured uterus in unrelieved obstruction – the fistula patients are the survivors.

The obstructed labour injury complex[1]

A fistula patient suffers from much more than a hole in the bladder. Her whole person is damaged. It is important to understand the full impact of the damage to the physical and mental well-being of the patient.

'Obstructed labour injury complex' is a term for a broad range of injuries that the patient suffering from an obstetric fistula may encounter. These can be divided into primary conditions directly due to the ischaemia from the obstructed labour and conditions that are secondary to this ischaemic damage.

Primary conditions

The predominant lesion
This is a communication between the vagina and urinary tract, always involving the bladder and often the urethra.

Recto-vaginal fistulae
Recto-vaginal fistulae (RVFs) may coexist with VVFs in more severe cases of ischaemia. The incidence of combined fistulae ranges from 5% to 10%. Isolated RVFs are rare.

Ureteric fistulae
Ureteric fistulae can arise in two ways:

- They can result from involvement of the uretero-vesical junction in the ischaemic process, so that the ureter then drains directly into the vagina away from the fistula margin.
- More often, they are caused by operative injury during caesarean section or an emergency hysterectomy for a ruptured uterus.

Renal damage
A few fistula patients develop a stricture of the lower ureter leading to hydronephrosis and loss of renal function.

Genital tract injuries
The ischaemic process may destroy the tissues of the vagina, cervix and even the uterus. This leads to degrees of vaginal stenosis, loss of the anterior cervix and canal, and occasionally severe cervical stenosis leading to haematometra. Exceptionally, the whole uterus sloughs.

Nerve damage
Many fistula patients suffer compression damage to the lumbo-sacral plexus. The most common manifestation is foot drop from involvement of the L5 root. Minor degrees are easily overlooked. About 90% of patients with foot drop do slowly recover, but this can take up to 2 years. In the most severe cases of pelvic ischaemia, the patient may be paraplegic immediately after delivery, but this too recovers (apart from prolonged foot drop). There may also be saddle anaesthesia with the loss of anal reflex and the risk of pressure sores.

Muscle and fascial damage
The levator muscles, especially the pubo-coccygeus, and the pelvic fascial support are subject to ischaemic damage when they are crushed against the inferior pubic rami.

Bone damage
In about 30% of cases of obstetric fistula, a pelvic X-ray will reveal damage to the region of the pubic symphysis.

Secondary conditions

Social consequences
The social consequences of obstetric fistula can be just as devastating to the patient as the symptoms of incontinence. Many women will be ostracized by their families and communities. Attitudes to fistula patients vary from region to region: in some areas, the family can be very supportive; however, the longer a woman has had a fistula, the more likely it is that her husband will divorce her. Many patients will be unable to socialize or to go to market, church or community gatherings, and will live a life of exclusion.

Mental health

It is not surprising that many fistula patients are severely depressed. A stillbirth followed by incontinence is too much to bear. One hundred per cent of patients in Ethiopia test positive for psychological disorder when questioned on arrival at the hospital, with up to 40% thinking seriously of suicide. Interestingly, 30% still test positive on leaving hospital, even though they are dry. Making the patient dry is not always the end of her problems.

Urine dermatitis

Many patients restrict their drinking and end up with very concentrated urine. When the patient is incontinent, the phosphates and nitrates contained in the urine irritate the skin, causing local hyperkeratosis and secondary ulceration. The cure is to treat the incontinence, but in the meantime the condition will improve if the patient can drink more and dilute her urine. Barrier substances such as petroleum jelly may help. Also, dilute urine does not smell nearly so much.

Bladder stones

Concentrated urine will predispose to deposits in the bladder that may act as a nidus for the formation of stones. These can become large and can cause pain, haematuria and odour from chronic cystitis.

Some women may have had a foreign body introduced into the bladder either by themselves or by a traditional healer in an effort to stop the flow of urine. Such objects include cloth, plant material and even small stones.

Contractures

Up to 2% of fistula patients in Ethiopia suffer severe lower limb contractures, although these are very rarely seen in other African countries. They occur after delivery, because the patient will often lie curled up in bed with her legs together, trying to stop the flow of urine. Patients may remain in this position for months or even years, resulting in diffuse contractures.

Malnutrition

In Ethiopia, in particular, neglect and depression lead to malnutrition in some patients, with a fall in body mass index (BMI). In contrast, this appears to be a less common problem in other tropical African countries.

Infertility

Many fistula patients (up to 60%) have amenorrhoea after delivery. This has a variety of causes, the main one being supratentorial, e.g. the severe mental stress of losing a child and a husband, together with the shame of incontinence. Malnutrition may also be a factor. A small number of patients will have Sheehan's syndrome – anterior pituitary necrosis due to prolonged shock during labour. The resultant decrease in follicle-stimulating hormone (FSH) and luteinizing hormone (LH) leads to amenorrhoea. Ashermann's syndrome – scarring of the endometrium by either repeated infections or perhaps urine in the endometrial cavity – is another cause.

These women may have normal hormone levels, but the endometrium will be unresponsive to them. Finally, there may be cryptomenorrhoea, or hidden menses, if the cervical canal is stenosed leading to haematometra.

Reproductive outcomes
For the above reasons, the potential for successful pregnancy in women with obstetric fistulae is quite low. Only about 20% of post-repair patients will achieve a term pregnancy. If a patient does become pregnant, she has a high chance of a miscarriage or prematurity. This is because of an incompetent cervix. The anterior lip is frequently torn so badly that it will not be strong enough to hold a pregnancy to term. Others have vaginal stenosis that is severe enough to preclude intercourse.

Other causes of incontinence not directly related to obstructed labour

In war-torn countries sexual violence is a tragic cause of genital tract injuries. The principles of management are the same as for obstetric fistulae.

Anyone working in developing countries will encounter some patients with miscellaneous causes of incontinence. These include:

- congenital abnormalities, including ectopia vesicae, epispadias and ectopic ureters (usually as part of a duplex system)
- neurological causes, such as spina bifida
- advanced carcinoma of the cervix
- ureteric fistulae produced during elective gynaecological operations
- genital prolapse conditions.

Management of these (apart from ureteric injuries) is outside the scope of this book.

Basis of classification of obstetric fistulae

Despite much debate, there is no universally accepted system of classification. This is understandable, because so much of the assessment is subjective. For a classification to be worthwhile, it should enable surgeons to communicate with each other and even consider clinical trials. Most surgeons base their classification on simple descriptive terms involving three factors:

- site
- size
- scarring.

Fistula site

Juxta-urethral
The most common site is juxta-urethral, i.e. at the urethro-vesical junction (Figures 1.3–1.5). In this situation, there is almost always loss of some proximal urethra. Mild

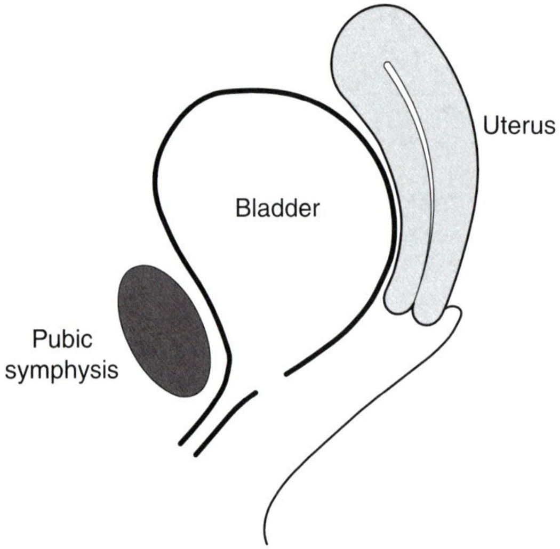

Figure 1.3 A simple juxta-urethral fistula.

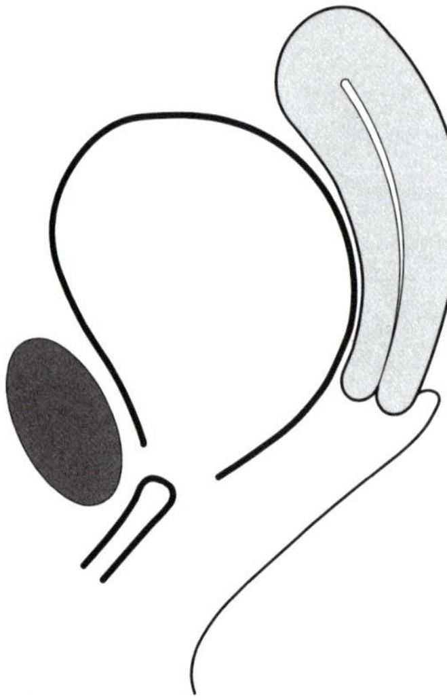

Figure 1.4 A small circumferential juxta-urethral fistula. There is a gap between the bladder and the urethra. The latter is often blocked.

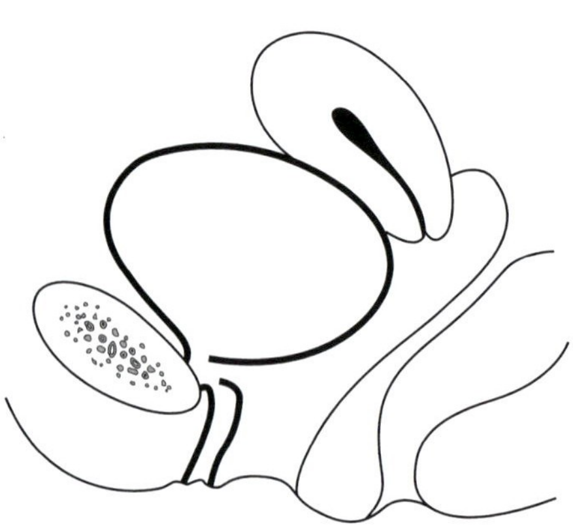

Figure 1.5 A circumferential juxta-urethral fistula is often pulled up and stuck to the back of the pubic symphysis, making it relatively inaccessible.

ischaemia will produce just a simple hole, but prolonged ischaemia will cause circumferential tissue loss with the urethra and bladder becoming separated to a variable extent.

Mid-vaginal

Small defects 4 cm or more from the external urethral orifice are not very common, but are very easy to repair. Larger defects may extend back as far as the cervix and laterally to the pubic rami.

Juxta-cervical

Juxta-cervical fistulae, i.e. fistulae in the region of the cervix (Figure 1.6), are common in multiparous patients and in those delivered by caesarean section. Patients who start to push before the cervix is fully dilated are prone to fistulae in this region. Sometimes, the defect extends into the cervical canal where the anterior cervical canal is completely missing or torn open (Figure 1.7). These fistulae presumably result from a vertical tear in the lower segment with associated bladder injury during caesarean section.

Intra-cervical

Intra-cervical fistulae, i.e. fistulae between the bladder and the cervical canal (Figure 1.8), are not very common. They almost always follow a caesarean section. There may be a history of a live baby, suggesting an iatrogenic cause.

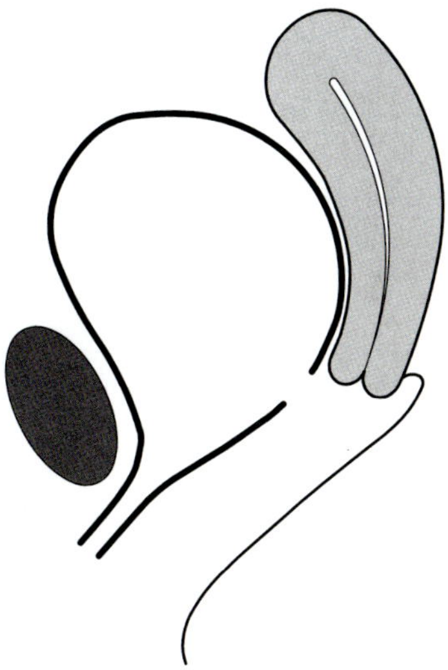

Figure 1.6 A simple juxta-cervical fistula.

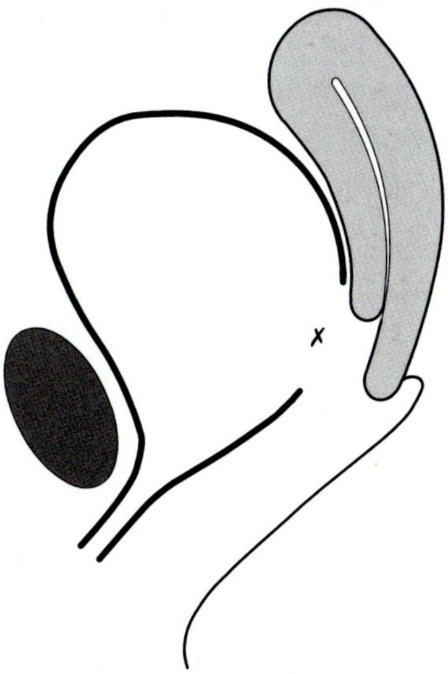

Figure 1.7 A juxta-cervical/intra-cervical fistula. The cross indicates the approximate position of the ureteric orifice.

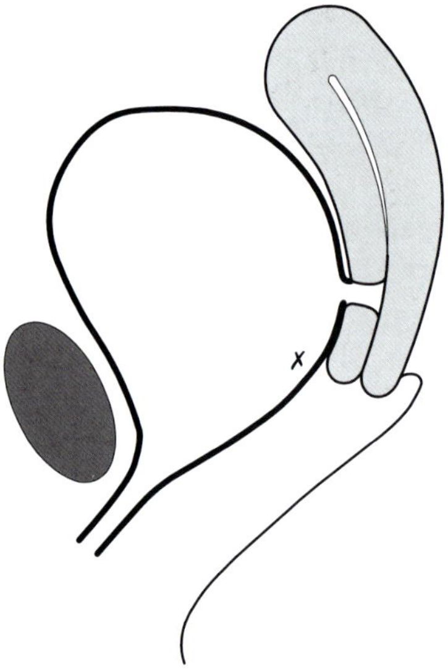

Figure 1.8 An intra-cervical fistula. The cross indicates the approximate position of the ureteric orifice.

Circumferential

The term 'circumferential fistula' is used when the bladder has been completely separated from the urethra (Figure 1.9). The urethra is almost always involved to some extent, and the extent of detachment varies from minimal with a normal-capacity bladder to extreme where the bladder has all but disappeared. The more common intermediate type is recognized clinically by palpation of bare bone at the back of the pubic symphysis. In these cases, most of the anterior vaginal wall and the base of bladder are destroyed.

Miscellaneous fistulae

Fistulae can result from accidental damage to a ureter during caesarean section or hysterectomy, and vault fistulae can be produced during emergency hysterectomy

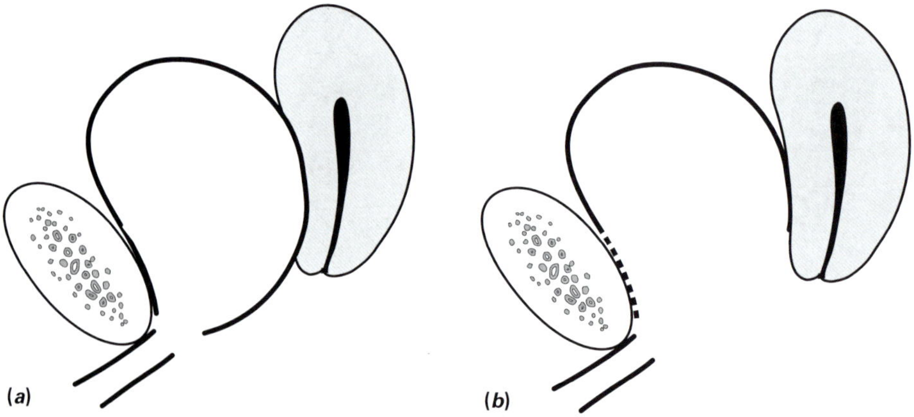

Figure 1.9 Circumferential fistulae: (*a*) small gap; (*b*) massive gap.

for a ruptured uterus or elective hysterectomy. Locally advanced carcinoma of the cervix can cause a urinary fistula.

Fistula size

Fistulae may be:

- tiny (admitting only a small probe)
- small (0.5–1.5 cm)
- medium (1.5–3 cm)
- large (>3 cm), usually involving loss of most of the anterior vaginal wall and a circumferential loss of the urethro-vesical junction
- extensive, i.e. involving major loss of bladder and urethra, with a large gap between the two (Figure 1.10).

Scarring

Scarring varies from minimal when the fistula margins are soft and mobile to extreme when the fistula margins are rigid and fixed. Scarring also affects the lateral and posterior wall of the vagina, causing complete stenosis in extreme cases. Vaginal stenosis can affect the proximal or distal canal or can extend throughout. The most common site is mid-vagina.

Scar is the big enemy – any fistula with significant scarring is not for a beginner.

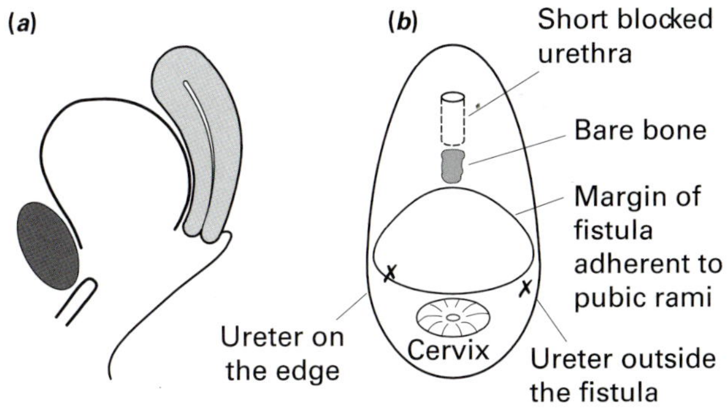

Figure 1.10 An extensive fistula: (*a*) sagittal section; (*b*) intra-vaginal view. The whole of the anterior vaginal wall has been lost; there is a gap between the stenosed urethra and the anterior bladder wall. Bare bone is exposed at the back of the pubic symphysis. The antero-lateral margins of the bladder defect are adherent to the underside of the pubic arch, and the ureteric openings will be on the edge or even outside the bladder, as indicated in (*b*).

Classification systems

Two recent attempts to standardize classification have been proposed, by Judith Goh and Kees Waaldijk.

Goh's system

Goh's classification[2] is based on three variables:

- the length of the urethra (types 1–4)
- the size of the fistula (a–c)
- the degree of scarring (I–III).

Urethral length

Type 1: Distal edge of fistula >3.5 cm from the external urethral orifice (EUO), i.e. the urethra is not involved

Type 2: Distal edge 2.5–3.5 cm from the EUO

Type 3: Distal edge 1.5–<2.5 cm from the EUO

Type 4: Distal edge <1.5 cm from the EUO.

Fistula size

(a) Size <1.5 cm

(b) Size 1.5–3 cm

(c) Size >3 cm.

Scarring

I. No or mild fibrosis around fistula/vagina, and/or vagina length >6 cm or normal capacity

II. Moderate or severe fibrosis around fistula and/or vagina, and/or reduced vaginal length and/or capacity

III. Special considerations, e.g. circumferential fistula, involvement of ureteric orifices.

We presently use this classification, as we believe it to be the best attempt to be objective about clinical findings. However, there are still problems with the system:

- The urethral length is often only estimated, but is important in predicting prognosis and management.
- Assessment of the degree of scarring and shortening of the vagina is inevitably subjective.

- There may be lack of agreement as to what constitutes a circumferential fistula. Even small juxta-urethral fistulae may be slightly detached from the bladder, although some surgeons reserve the term 'circumferential' for cases where there is a clearly palpable gap with bare bone between the urethra and the bladder.
- The ureteric orifices may be just inside, at the edge of or outside the fistula, so ureteric involvement is open to subjective interpretation.

Thus, there may be considerable inter-observer variation; however, if a surgeon applies the same criteria in all cases, this will enable a meaningful audit to be done.

As an example, we have used this classification to confirm our suspicion that the worst fistulae occur in primiparous patients and those having a vaginal delivery (see Appendix 2).

This system of grading from type 1aI to type 4cIII does indicate an increasingly poor prognosis, although it is not always an indication of difficulty of repair. Type 1aI cases have the best prognosis and are often the easiest to repair, but a small inaccessible fistula high in the vagina or cervical canal would have the same classification but might be a great challenge to close.

In addition, the surgeon should make an estimate of bladder size. This is done with a calibrated sound at the beginning of the operation. An additional refinement is to measure functional bladder capacity during dye testing.

Waaldijk's system

The classification proposed in Waaldijk's book[3] has been valuable in predicting outcome and planning treatment, and has been vital for his own analysis of outcomes. It has not been universally adopted, but it is used by the many surgeons whom he has trained.

Type I: Fistulae ≥5 cm from the EUO and therefore not involving the closing mechanism. These have an excellent prognosis, because the all-important urethra and bladder neck are intact.

Type II: Fistulae that involve the closing mechanism (<5cm from the EUO):

A. Without (sub)total involvement of the urethra:

(a) without a circumferential defect

(b) with a circumferential defect

B. With (sub)total involvement of the urethra:

(a) without a circumferential defect

(b) with a circumferential defect.

Type III: Miscellaneous fistulae, e.g. uretero-vaginal and other exceptional fistulae.

Some surgeons have had difficulty in distinguishing between types IIA and IIB, although recently Waaldijk (personal communication) has clarified this by defining type IIB fistulae as those with a urethral remnant of less than 1.5 cm.

A descriptive template

In reality, each fistula case is unique, and there are so many variables that some surgeons feel that a satisfactory classification will never be achieved. To a large extent, the description of fistulae and their repair can be learned only by long apprenticeship. We recommend the use of a simple template for figurative description of clinical findings and operative details. This is very helpful in communication between individual surgeons. One such template, based on that used at the Addis Ababa Fistula Hospital, is illustrated in Figure 1.11, where the fistula is indicated roughly in size and in its position in relation to the urethra and cervix. The amount of shading indicates the degree of scarring in the vagina or around the fistula margins.

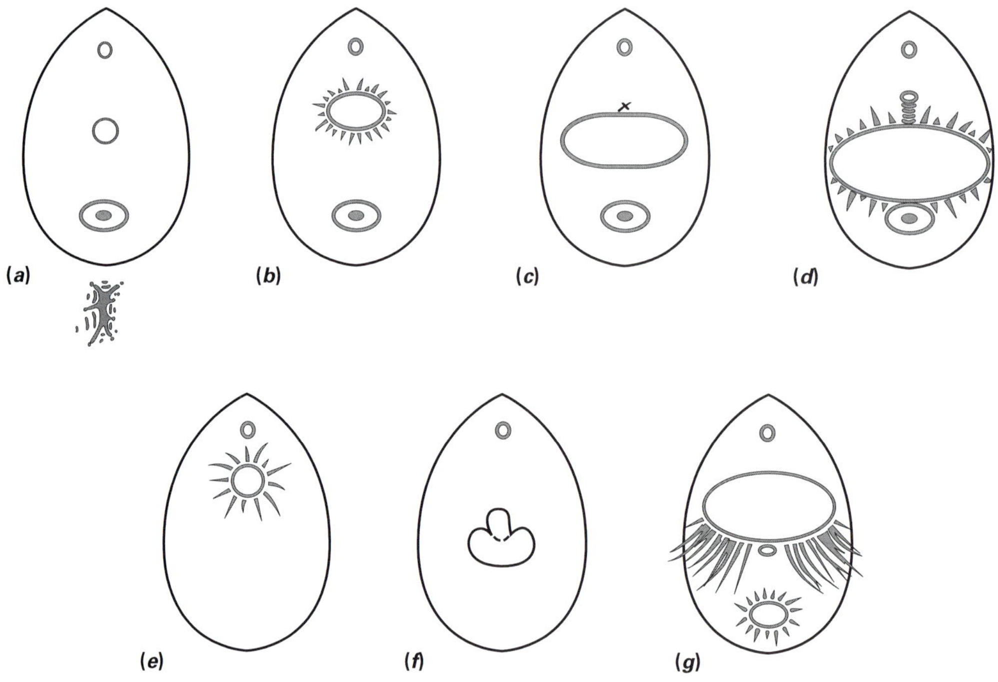

Figure 1.11 (*a*) A simple small mid-vaginal vesico-vaginal fistula (VVF). (*b*) A medium VVF with some scarring of the margins. (*c*) A larger VVF without scarring but with a blocked urethra. (*d*) A large circumferential VVF with severe scarring and a gap between the urethra and the bladder. (*e*) Severe vaginal stenosis. (*f*) A juxta-cervical fistula extending into an open cervical canal. (*g*) A large VVF with severe posterior scarring of the vagina and a recto-vaginal fistula as well.

Prognosis

The critical factors affecting the prognosis of an obstetric fistula are the length of the urethra, the sizes of the fistula and the bladder, and the amount of scarring. Almost all defects can be closed (although bladder capacity may be reduced). However, if the urethra has been crushed, denervated and shortened, it will not function and the patient may have total stress incontinence. The shorter the urethra and the greater the scarring, the higher is the chance of stress incontinence. Destroyed urethras can be repaired, but the prognosis for continence is not good.

References

1. Arrowsmith S, Hamlin C, Wall L. Obstetric labour injury complex: obstetric fistula formation and the multifaceted morbidity of maternal birth trauma in the developing world. CME review article. *Obstet Gynecol Surv* 1996; **51**: 568–74.
2. Goh JWT, Krause HG. *Female Genital Tract Fistula.* Brisbane: University of Queensland Press, 2004.
3. Waaldijk K. *Step by Step Surgery of Vesico-Vaginal Fistulas.* Edinburgh: Campion Press, 1994.

2 Diagnosis

History taking

The following details are required:

- **Symptoms**. It should be confirmed that the patient is wet all the time. If she is dry at night then she probably does not have a fistula (although there are exceptions – see 'Dye test' below). She should be asked whether there is any leakage of faeces as well as urine. A small hole in the bladder leaks just as much as a large one, but some patients with a rectal fistula may only be aware of soiling when they have diarrhoea.
- **Age.**
- **Parity**. If the patient is multiparous then which delivery caused the fistula?
- **How long has the patient been wet?**
- **Mode of delivery.** Was birth by vaginal delivery or caesarean section?
- **How long was she in labour?** The average is about 3 days.
- **Where did the delivery take place**? Home, maternity centre or hospital?
- **Did the child survive?** Almost all vaginal deliveries result in a stillbirth, but a few delivered by caesarean section are alive. This strongly suggests an iatrogenic injury.
- **Neurological symptoms.** Complete paralysis is rare, but minor degrees of foot drop are common.
- **Does she still menstruate?** Amenorrhoea is quite common after such a traumatic childbirth, but if the patient had a caesarean section then one should suspect a hysterectomy for a ruptured uterus. Some patients do not know that they have lost their uterus.
- **Have any attempts been made to repair the fistula**? Patients sometimes hide this information for fear that they will be turned away.
- **Social history.** The majority of patients with a long-standing fistula are single and live a very restricted life. The longer that they have had the fistula, the more likely it is that they will be alone and live a subsistence existence supported by relatives.

History taking does not help very much in selecting the easy cases. There are, however, some clues that should arouse suspicion of a serious injury:

- Neurological weakness (usually foot drop), even if it has recovered, is indicative of this.
- Rectal fistulae are usually associated with a serious bladder injury. This does not apply to anal sphincter injuries, which often occur in isolation and should not be classified as recto-vaginal fistulae.
- Fistulae following a caesarean section are often in the region of the cervix, owing to a combination of ischaemia and operative trauma.
- A fistula following hysterectomy for a ruptured uterus will usually be in the vault or due to an accidental ureteric injury.

Examination

Inspection

The abdomen

Are caesarean or other scars present? Is any swelling visible? The patient could be pregnant! Repair should generally be avoided in pregnancy unless it is the patient's only real chance of finding a skilled surgeon. Bleeding can be very troublesome during the repair.

The perineum

- Look for obvious wetness and urine dermatitis (Figure 2.1). (The dermatitis is caused by concentrated urine. The patient should be asked to drink more if it is not possible to operate immediately.)
- Can the urethral orifice be seen? In very bad fistulae, it can be completely destroyed (Figure 2.2).

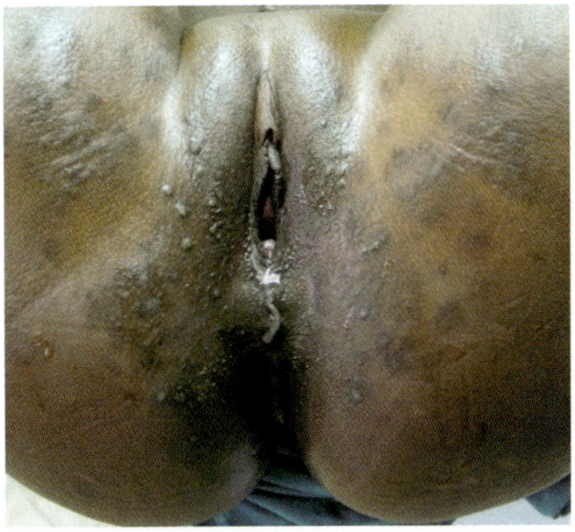

Figure 2.1 Urine dermatitis.

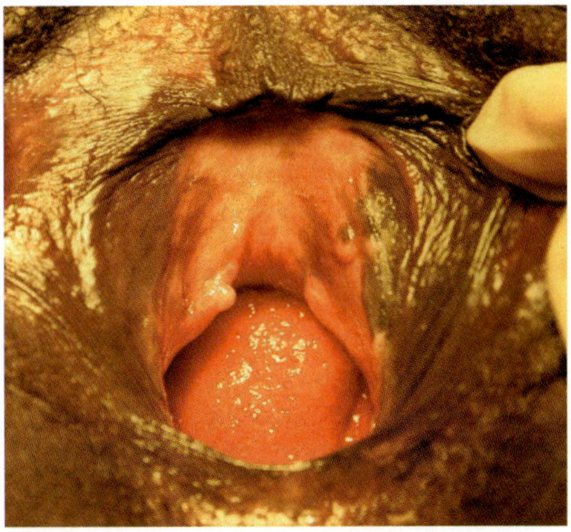

Figure 2.2 A case with complete destruction of the urethra and the prolapsed bladder filling the vagina.

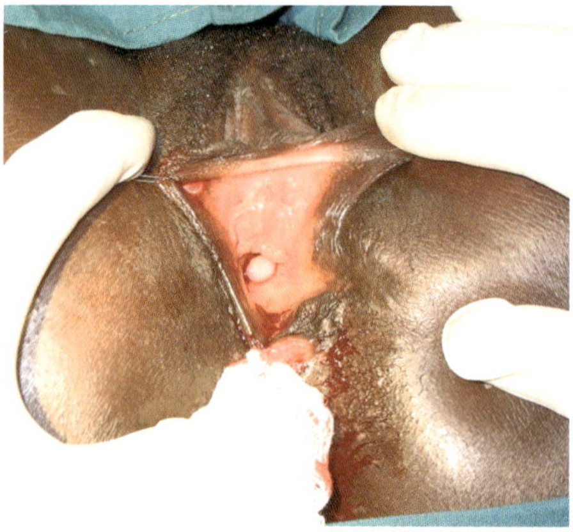

Figure 2.3 A superficial stenosis seen on inspection.

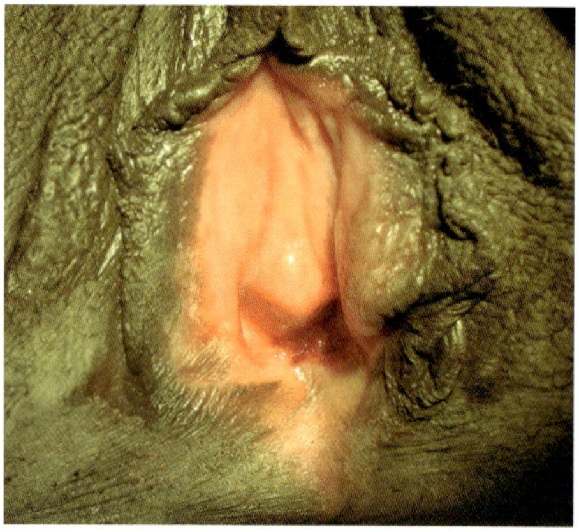

Figure 2.4 Complete dense occlusion of the vagina.

- Is there any sign of stenosis (Figures 2.3 and 2.4)?

Palpation

Begin with the abdomen in order to exclude an unexpected pregnancy or other swellings. Follow this with a vaginal examination. Use the lubricated index finger gently.

- Is the vagina of normal size and depth? Can the cervix be felt? Is there any vaginal narrowing? Smaller degrees are felt as a band of fibrous tissue around the lateral and posterior circumference at any depth in the vagina. In extreme cases, the whole vagina is stenosed. The anterior wall is frequently shortened in the presence of a fistula. Carefully palpate the posterior wall for a recto-vaginal fistula.
- Can a defect be felt in the anterior vaginal wall? This will range from a large defect where the finger immediately enters the bladder, to smaller defects that just admit a finger, to the smallest ones where no defect is felt at all. If a defect can be felt, where is it in relation to the urethra and the cervix? If a defect can be felt, consider the margins carefully. Are they soft and supple, somewhat rigid or (in the worst cases) stuck to the pubic rami?
- The anterior cervix is often torn in fistula patients. Defects in this region are often difficult to feel unless they are large. The cervix may be easily felt low down in the vagina when a large amount of anterior wall has been lost.
- Feel the posterior vaginal wall carefully for a rectal defect. Rectal fistulae are usually associated with severe vaginal scarring and a bad bladder fistula, but occasionally they are small, soft and easily overlooked or just hidden behind a posterior band of scar. If one is suspected, a rectal examination should also be performed. Look at the perineal body and anal sphincters for any tears.

If preferred, the fistula can be inspected. This is best done with the patient in the lithotomy position using a Sims speculum, although some surgeons prefer the left lateral position with the right leg supported.

What should be done if the patient says that she is wet but it is not possible to see any wetness or feel a fistula?

In this situation, the patient should be asked to drink plenty and then be re-examined. (It should be remembered that many patients drink very little, especially if they know that they are going to be examined.) If it is then confirmed that the patient is wet but the fistula cannot be felt, proceed as follows:

- With the patient in the left lateral position, use a Sims speculum to expose the anterior vaginal wall (Figure 2.5). Ask the patient to cough. A small fistula may be readily visible.
- Alternatively, perform a dye test in this position or the position shown in Figure 2.6.

Dye test (Figure 2.6)

Dilute methylene blue (or gentian violet) should be used – if it is too concentrated, it will stain everything, making interpretation of the test difficult.

1. Insert a catheter.
2. Fill the catheter balloon with dye and have two or three moist swabs ready to put into the vagina.
3. Insert the swabs well into the vagina.
4. Slowly instil about 60 cm^3 of dye.

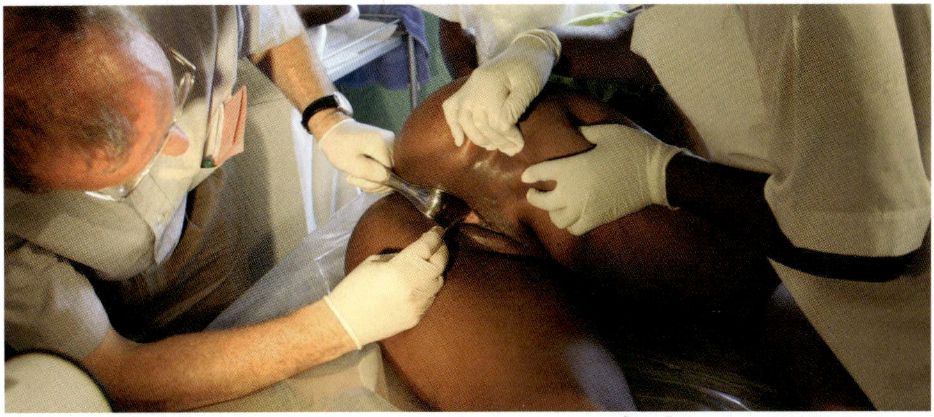

Figure 2.5 Exposure of the anterior vaginal wall.

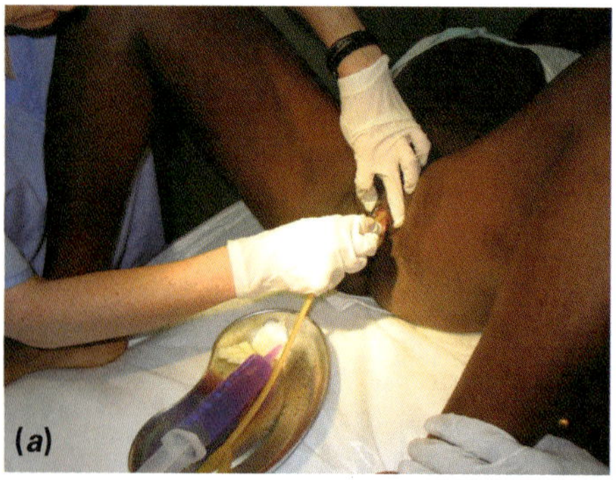

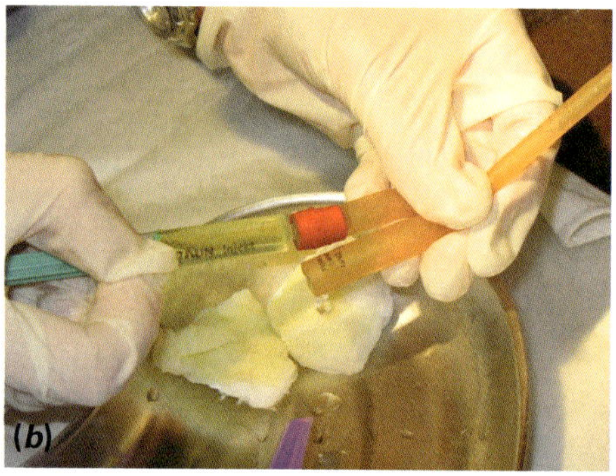

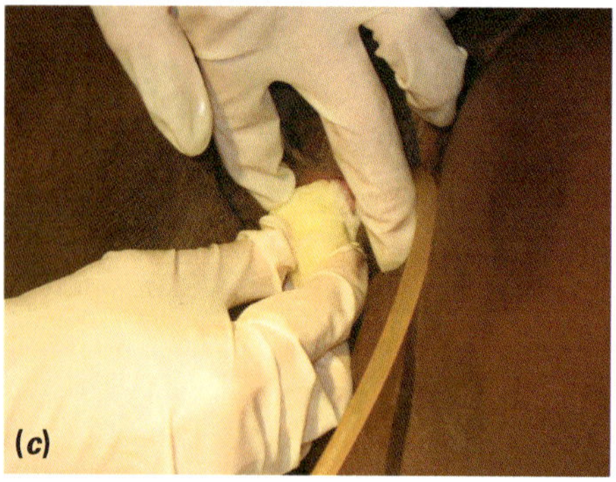

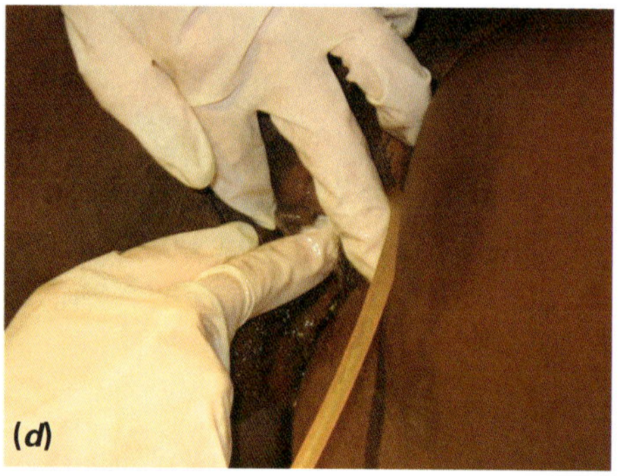

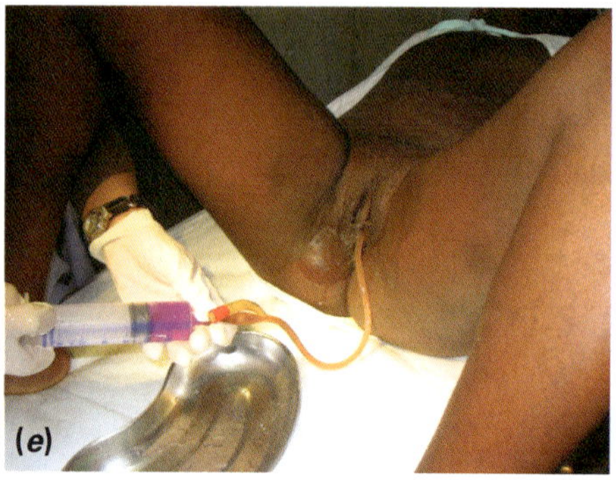

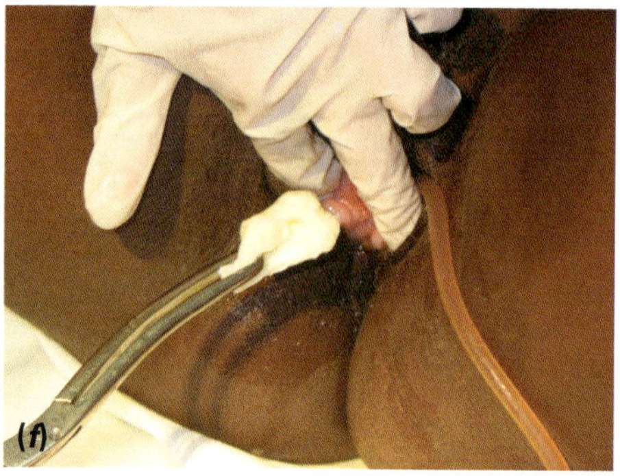

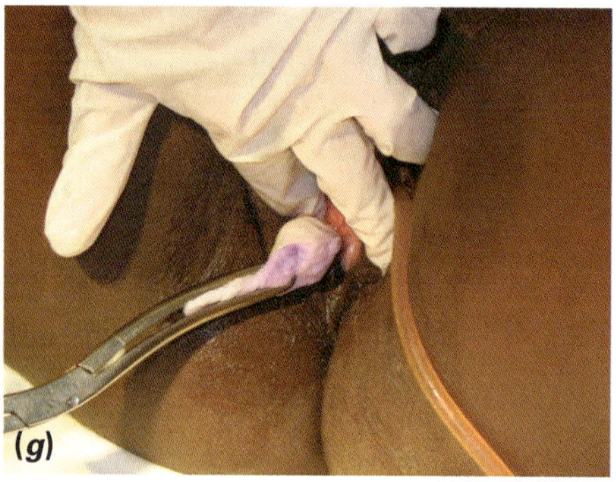

Figure 2.6 Dye test. (*a*) Insertion of catheter. (*b*) The balloon of the catheter is inflated, and two or three moist swabs are readied to be put into the vagina. (*c, d*) The swabs are inserted well into the vagina. (*e*) About 60 cm^3 of dye are slowly instilled. (*f, g*) The swabs are removed one by one: the first is not stained, but the second is stained blue, confirming that there is a fistula.

5. After 1 minute, ask the patient to cough.
6. Remove the swabs one by one.
7. If any of the swabs are stained, this indicates the presence of a fistula.
8. If none of the swabs is stained, there could still be a fistula. Repeat the test using up to 200 cm^3 of dye. The patient should walk around for 20 minutes while the dye is in the bladder. Sometimes the hole is very small, especially if it is between the cervix and the bladder. It is easy to overlook a tiny fistula.
9. If this second test is negative but the swab is wet with urine, there is a ureteric fistula.

Ureteric fistulae

A ureter can be damaged accidentally during a caesarean section, but injury is more likely during an emergency hysterectomy for a ruptured uterus. The ureter may be ligated and included in the lower-segment repair. Later, urine starts leaking through the cervix. After hysterectomy, urine may leak into the pelvis, and some days later finds a way out between the sutures in the vaginal vault. Although ureteric fistulae are uncommon, it is very important to recognize them, because they can be easily repaired by an abdominal operation (see Chapter 6).

To exclude a ureteric fistula, empty the bladder and insert a dry swab into the vagina. Ask the patient to drink and walk about. Re-examine her after half an hour. If the swab is wet then there is a ureteric fistula. On questioning, the patient should admit to being able to empty her bladder, as the other ureter should be functioning normally.

Postpartum stress and chronic retention

Postpartum stress is occasionally troublesome, and can be mistaken for a fistula. Following the dye test, take the catheter out, leaving the dye inside. Watch to see if it dribbles out of the urethra, and then ask the patient to cough. If there is significant stress, dye will come out. Then check her residual urine after voiding. Management is conservative with pelvic floor exercises, but surgery is occasionally needed after at least 6 months of conservative management.

Another uncommon cause of incontinence is the postpartum atonic bladder leading to overflow incontinence. Bladder function is disturbed by prolonged labour. This condition should be managed prophylactically by continuous bladder drainage post delivery for at least 8–10 days. If this is not done, chronic retention may result and be diagnosed much later when it is hard to treat. It may settle after a period of continuous catheter drainage, although a better option is to teach the patient intermittent self-catheterization.

Investigations

These include the following:

- Haemoglobin.
- Ultrasound scan. If available, this should be used more often, especially for bad cases. It is useful to be forewarned of a dilated renal tract.
- Intravenous urograms. These are rarely available, but can give useful information about the function of the kidneys when ureteric involvement is suspected.

3 Management of Early Cases

Conservative management

After a caesarean section for prolonged obstructed labour, the catheter should be retained for at least 10 days. Earlier removal predisposes to chronic retention. The bladder is often atonic after a prolonged labour. If there is urinary leakage after removal of the catheter, it should be reinserted immediately.

Initially, a defect will probably not be visible, because it will be out of sight in the region of the cervix and because of slough. The patient should be kept on continuous drainage, provided that most of the urine is coming through the catheter. After 2 or 3 weeks, it should be possible to assess the size of the defect by palpation and inspection. Up to 20–40% of small defects (<2 cm) may still heal with another 2–3 weeks of bladder drainage.

After vaginal delivery, a leak of urine may indicate anything from a tiny hole to massive necrosis. The patient should be examined gently with a Sims speculum. Slough should be seen; it must not be pulled or cut. Only if it is loose can it be gently pulled out (Figure 3.1). This should be followed by regular irrigation of the vagina. Palpation and inspection with a Sims speculum will help to judge the size of the fistula. If it is less than 2 cm in diameter, the catheter should be kept in at least another 4 weeks. It is difficult to keep the catheter in the bladder in the case of a larger fistula. Always check by vaginal examination that the catheter has not gone through the fistula into the vagina.

Fistulae that have not healed spontaneously with 4 weeks of drainage are unlikely to do so.

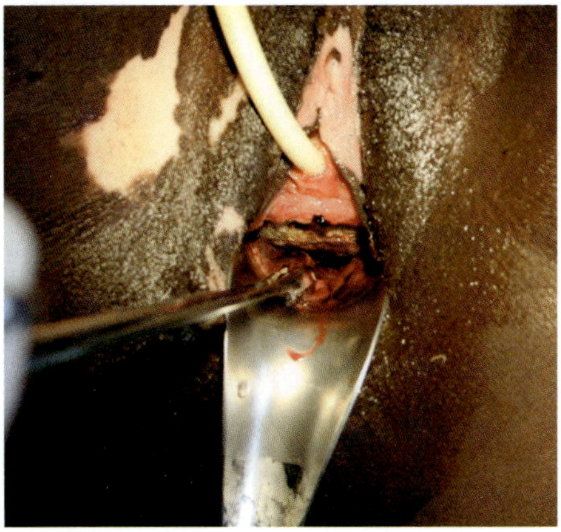

Figure 3.1 Slough should be removed only if really loose. This is not ready.

Note that antibiotics have no part to play in the healing of fistulae. The cause is ischaemic necrosis, not infection.

Prevention at caesarean section

In Uganda, two-thirds of patients with fistulae have had their obstructed labour relieved by caesarean section – but clearly too late. The remaining one-third have eventually delivered vaginally. In other countries, the incidence of caesarean section may be different. In Ethiopia, only 15% of fistula patients have had a caesarean section, because most people live in remote areas far from any hospital.

The ischaemic damage may already have occurred by the time of the caesarean section, but the doctor can take steps to minimize any further damage. The lower segment will be very stretched and unhealthy. Remember that the bladder should be dissected well down off the lower segment. The incision in the lower segment should be on the high side and the lateral ends curved upwards to minimize inaccessible tears (the left ureter is most at risk when repairing a lower segment).

When the baby's head is deeply impacted in the pelvis, it is better to get help to push up the head vaginally than to force a hand down between the head and the lower segment. This may produce vertical tears and increase the damage already done. The alternative is to extract the baby as a breech birth if possible.

Tears in the lower segment can be difficult to suture, and sometimes fistulae are produced when the doctor inadvertently picks up the bladder. This produces an intra-cervical fistula that can be quite a challenge to close and is not for the beginner. Ureters are at risk in difficult operations.

Are too many caesarean sections being performed for dead babies? In Uganda, 88% of mothers who develop fistulae after a caesarean section have a stillbirth. In the 12% with live babies, there is a strong suspicion of iatrogenic injury to the ureter or bladder.

A generation ago, it was commonplace to recommend a craniotomy for a dead baby stuck in the pelvis, but this seems to have been abandoned. It is not practised in teaching hospitals; perhaps it is too difficult for many young doctors to develop the skill. A craniotomy performed badly may do more harm than good. Is it time to look again at this procedure? This is something that only obstetricians working in the developing world can answer.

Early repair

Naturally, the sooner a patient can be cured the better. The longer she is incontinent, the greater is the chance that she will be abandoned. This is almost inevitable when she perceives that there is no chance of cure.

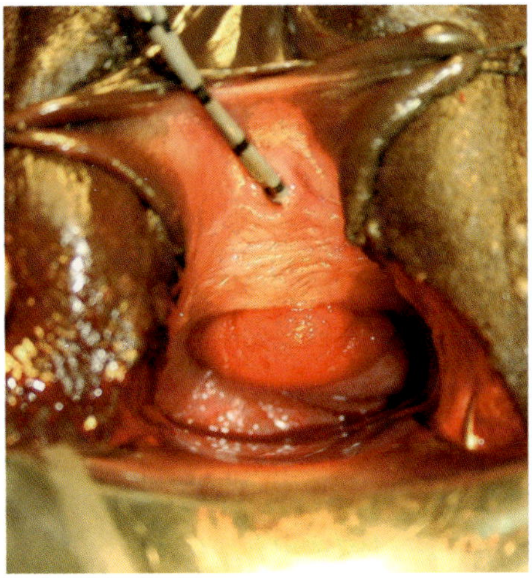

Figure 3.2 This fistula is only 2 months old, but is clean and suitable for repair.

Most surgeons advise waiting at least 3 months from the injury before operating. In the early months, the surrounding tissues are oedematous and hyperaemic, making them friable and difficult to handle. By 3 months, they should be sufficiently mature.

In spite of this, some surgeons have been very successful in closing selected fistulae before 3 months and have strongly recommended this approach.[1] Excellent results have been published, but the method has not yet been well illustrated or widely understood. We have not yet been able to reproduce such good results.

We have adopted a flexible approach in which each case is judged on its merits. Some fistulae are perfectly clean and healthy at 2 months, and can be safely repaired (Figure 3.2); on the other hand, some are distinctly friable even at 3 months. It is the appearance of the fistula that matters more than its age. If in doubt, wait.

We recommend that a beginner follow traditional advice and delay repair for 3 months. The first repair always has the best chance of success, and this should not be compromised. After some experience has been gained, exceptions can be made to this rule.

Reference

1. Waaldijk K. The immediate management of fresh obstetric fistulas. *Am J Obstet Gynecol* 2004; **191**: 795–9.

4 Preoperative Preparation

Is the patient fit for operation?

In Uganda, we find that most patients are in good general condition and ready for operation after a day's preparation. In Ethiopia, more patients are weak and malnourished, and a few have contractures. Findings will vary from country to country. It is always advisable to improve the patient's general condition by improved nutrition, iron and vitamin supplements, de-worming, and treatment of malaria. Contractures should be treated before surgery if possible.

Haemoglobin should be estimated. It should ideally be above 10 g/100 mL, but lower levels can be accepted for simple cases, where blood loss should be minimal. For difficult cases, blood should be taken for grouping. Transfusion is occasionally advisable.

It is not surprising that a recent small study has confirmed that many patients suffer from severe depression. Sympathetic handling is called for, but no amount of 'counselling' will improve a patient's mental state until she has been cured of constant incontinence.

Neurological damage and physiotherapy

Neurological damage is a marker for a severe injury. At the extreme, the patient may be unable to walk immediately after delivery due to ischaemia to the lumbar–sacral plexus (Figure 4.1). Immobility may lead to pressure sores, compounded by the presence of saddle anaesthesia.

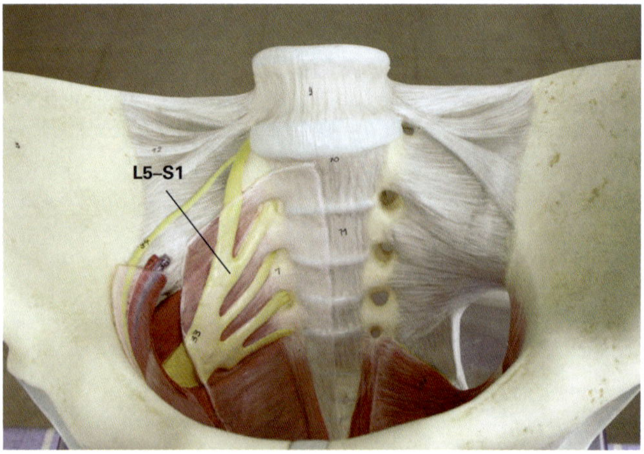

Figure 4.1 The L5–S1 roots are particularly at risk from ischaemia at the pelvic inlet.

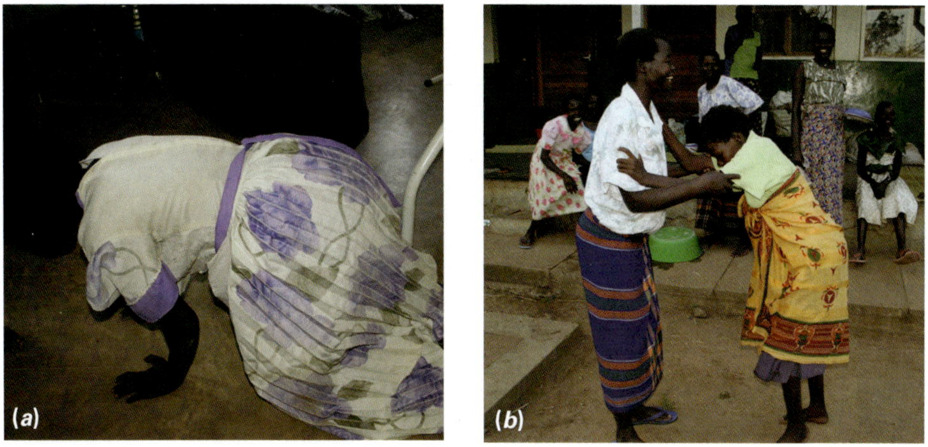

Figure 4.2 (*a*) This patient could only crawl 2 weeks post delivery. She has both a vesico-vaginal fistula and a recto-vaginal fistula. (*b*) One week later, she could just walk with support, but had bilateral foot drop. At 6 months, she just had mild unilateral foot drop. Both fistulae were closed, but stress incontinence remained a problem.

With good nursing care, the majority of patients improve (Figure 4.2). With good nutrition and active and passive movements of all joints, motor power and sensory loss will improve, although foot drop (due to damage to the L5 root) will be the last to recover (if it does at all). The provision of splints prevents contractures in plantar flexion. However, they should not be a substitute for putting all affected joints through a full range of movement several times daily. Residual foot drop, especially if a fixed plantar flexion has been allowed to develop, is a serious disability that will impair the patient's ability in daily activities.

It is easy to understand how, in the absence of any medical help, contractures form, especially if the patient is rejected and lies in one position for days on end, hoping that the incontinence will stop (Figure 4.3). This is particularly prone to occur in Ethiopian society, where many of the patients are child brides in remote areas. About 2% of patients presenting at the Addis Ababa Fistula Hospital have severe contractures. These require months of passive stretching exercises before they are fit for repair. A dedicated physiotherapy department enables severe contractures to be considerably improved in time (Figure 4.4).

Explanation

Clearly, the patient must be prepared for what is going to happen in the operating theatre and must give her consent. She must be informed about the length of postoperative stay, the duration the catheter will be kept in and the restrictions on her activities. She and her attendant must understand that they should not rush off home immediately the catheter is removed. Those who operate on difficult cases

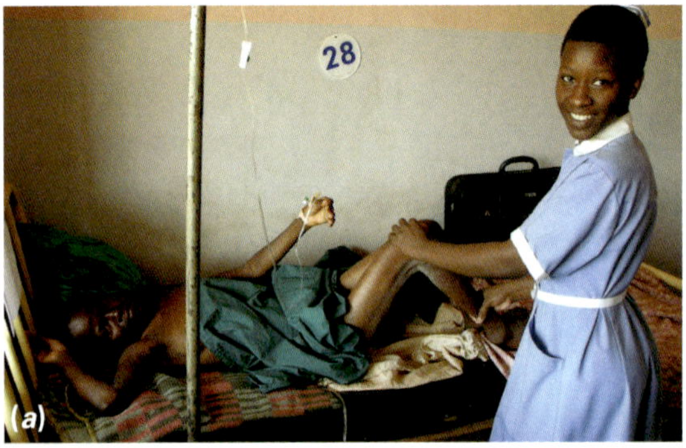

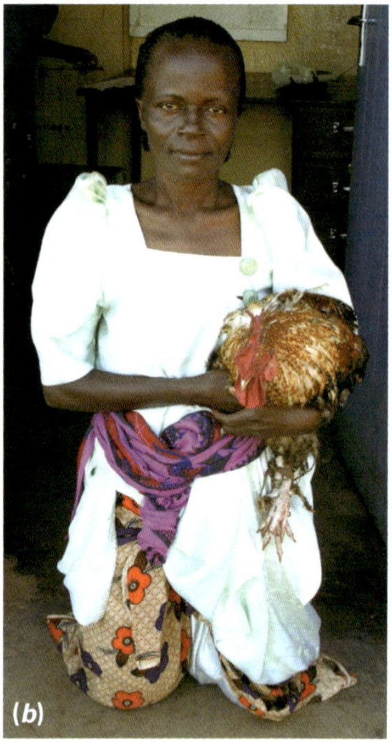

Figure 4.3 (*a*) This was the only patient in over 1000 seen in Uganda who had significant contractures. She had lived in a sack for 6 months after her stillbirth! There was no time to correct the contractures, so her fistula was repaired. (*b*) She returned cured of her incontinence, bearing a chicken in thanks, but still walking on her knees. In spite of careful instruction, she had been unable to find anyone to help her with regular stretching exercises after her operation.

would be wise to warn the patient of the limitations of surgery in achieving a cure, including the risk of stress incontinence, so that expectations are not raised too high.

Bowel preparation

It is best to have the rectum empty during the operation in case there is any leakage though the anus. In ideal circumstances, the patient would have an enema the day before, but in reality enemas are forgotten or given at the last minute, often leading to contamination during the operation. It is much better to give no enema at all and simply to be sure that the patient has been asked to open her bowels before coming to theatre.

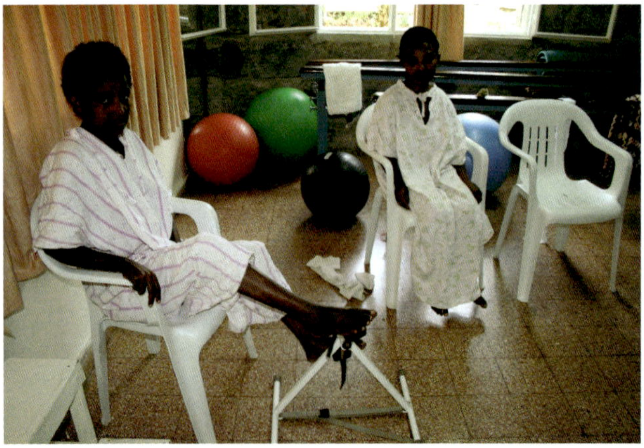

Figure 4.4 The Addis Ababa Fistula Hospital has a well-equipped physiotherapy department. Months of work must be done to slowly improve contractures.

An enema does need to be given the evening before operation in cases of recto-vaginal fistula or sphincter repair.

In the uncommon event of troublesome anal leakage, we clean up and insert a temporary anal purse-string suture, and carry on operating.

Hydration

Left to her own devices, the patient will come to theatre dehydrated, as she will be trying to reduce the amount of wetness. This is a bad thing, for a number of reasons:

- She may be hypotensive under a spinal anaesthetic.
- It increases the difficulty in identifying the ureteric orifices.
- The urine output will be poor after the operation, predisposing to catheter blockage. More intravenous fluids will be required during and after the operation. They are expensive.

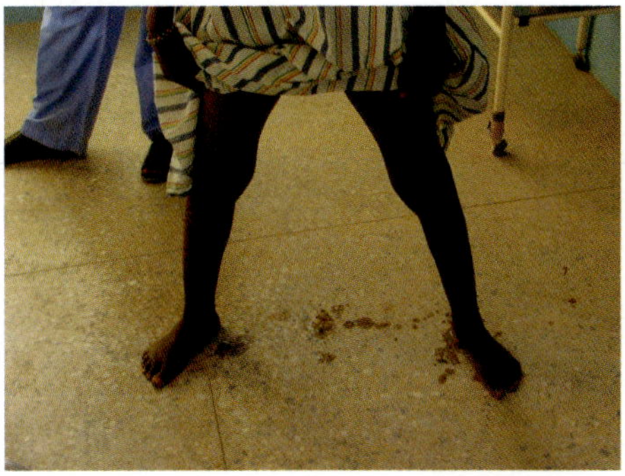

Figure 4.5 If the patient has been drinking sufficiently, urine should be seen dripping when she stands with her legs apart. (Photograph courtesy of Kees Waaldijk.)

Therefore, as soon as the decision is made to operate, ask the patient to start drinking plenty of mixed fluids, only stopping 4 hours before the operation. If she has been drinking sufficiently, urine should drip when she stands with her legs apart (Figure 4.5). Set up an intravenous infusion of saline before she goes to theatre,

Be aware of the very rare but serious condition of hyponatraemia (see Chapter 11).

5 In Theatre

The anaesthetic

Spinal anaesthesia is the preferred method for all fistula cases (Figure 5.1). Many surgeons give spinal anaesthesia themselves. Bupivacaine 0.5% in glucose (Marcain Heavy) is ideal as the longest-acting anaesthetic, although lidocaine 5% in glucose 7.5% can have its duration extended by the addition of adrenaline (epinephrine). The technique favoured by some is to draw up adrenaline 1 in 1000 into the syringe, expel it and then draw up the lidocaine. The wetting of the inside of the syringe provides enough adrenaline.

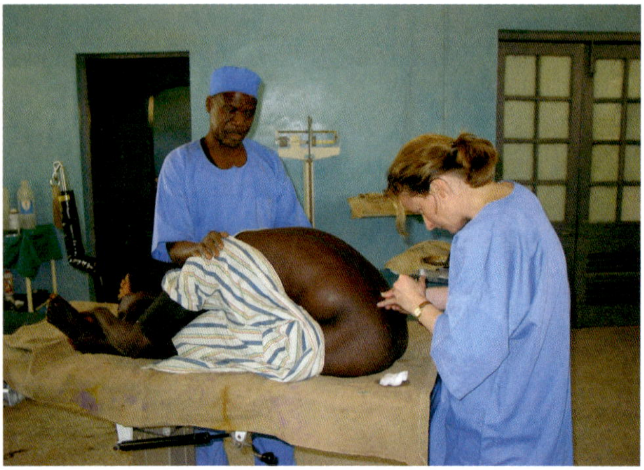

Figure 5.1 The ideal position in which to administer spinal anaesthesia. (Photograph taken at Katsina, courtesy of Kees Waaldijk.)

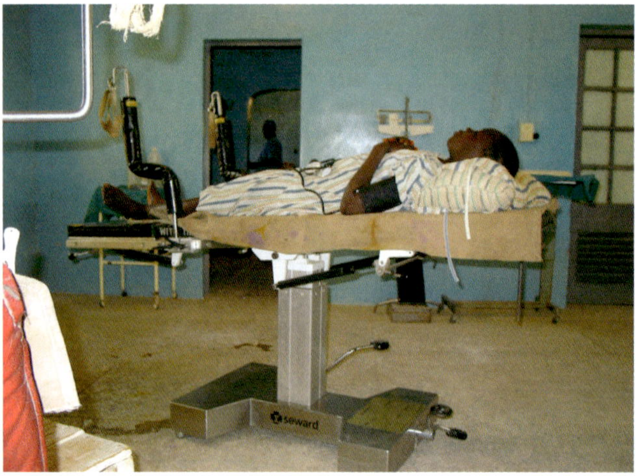

Figure 5.2 A slight head-up position with the head on a pillow is maintained for 10 minutes after the injection. (Photograph taken at Katsina, courtesy of Kees Waaldijk.)

The usual dose is 2 cm^3 of lidocaine 5% in glucose 7.5% or 2 cm^3 of Marcain Heavy. Some surgeons sit the patient up for 5 minutes; others lie the patient down, slightly head-up, for 5 minutes before putting the legs up; yet others lay the patient down and put the legs up in stirrups right away. The critical step is that there should be *no head-down tilt for at least 10 minutes* until all the anaesthetic has been fixed – otherwise paralysis of the respiratory centre may be fatal (Figure 5.2).

Both Kees Waaldijk and Andrew Browning, through force of circumstances, operate without any anaesthetic back-up, and can finish their operation before the spinal anaesthetic wears off. However, neither is able to perform any abdominal operations. Less experienced surgeons would not feel comfortable operating without anaesthetic help. Some patients require pethidine or occasionally ketamine to complete the operation, and unexpected emergencies can arise at any time.

Other surgeons, including myself, prefer the option of occasionally changing to an abdominal approach after assessment vaginally under spinal anaesthesia. If the patient was lying flat initially for 5 minutes, the spinal anaesthesia should be high enough to allow a lower abdominal approach, but it is essential to have anaesthetic back-up in case of difficulties during an abdominal operation.

Antibiotics

Some surgeons give no antibiotics, whereas a few prescribe them throughout the postoperative period.

It is well known that infection usually results from contamination during the operation, so it is our practice to give a single intravenous dose of gentamicin 160 mg at the start of surgery.

We would continue with antibiotics for 24 hours only if there has been accidental faecal contamination of a repair or if a rectal repair has also been performed. Our choice would be intramuscular gentamicin 80 mg and intravenous metronidazole 500 mg 8-hourly.

Instruments

Basic instruments

For simple fistulae, the following instruments are needed (Figure 5.3):

- Auvard speculum
- high-quality dissecting scissors
- toothed dissecting forceps
- Allis tissue forceps
- artery forceps

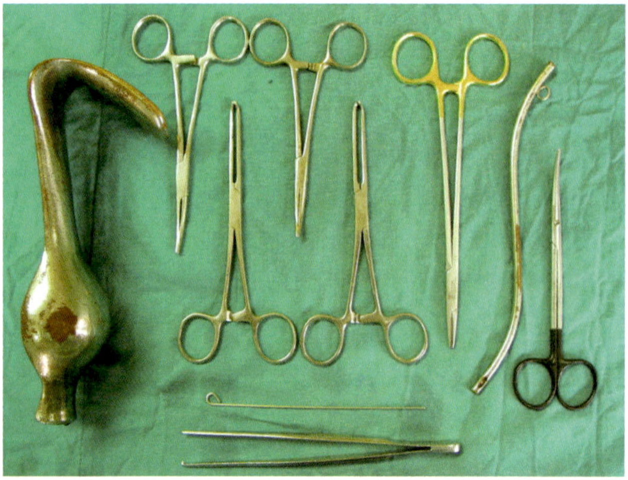

Figure 5.3 Basic instruments for a simple repair.

- metal catheter
- small probe
- no. 15 blade (not illustrated).

Additional instruments

For the full range of fistula surgery, some more specialized instruments are helpful.

Retractors

- Sims speculum for exposing the interior of the bladder
- small Langenbeck retractor for access to the vaginal fornices
- Auvard speculum – ideally, this should be available with short and long vaginal blades and with different angulations.

Scissors

Most surgeons have their favourite scissors; ours are the following (Figure 5.4):

- Boyd–Stille tonsil scissors for fine dissection
- Thorek scissors, sharply curved at the tip
- Stille–Matarasso fistula scissors for cutting through scar.

(See Appendix A for suppliers.)

Sutures and needles (Figure 5.5)

Non-absorbable sutures must never be used, because a stone may later form in the bladder.

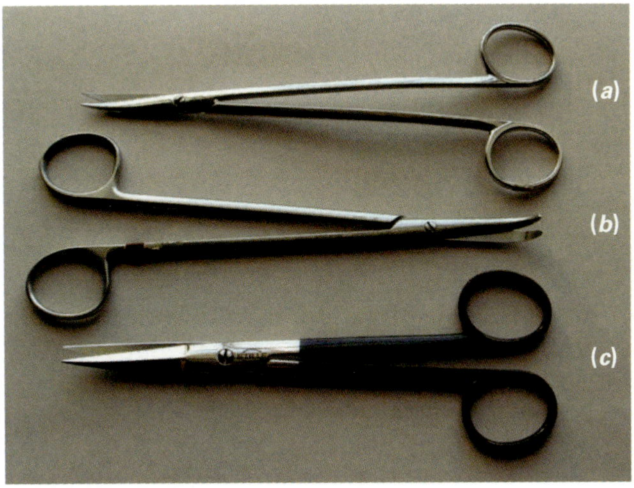

Figure 5.4 Scissors: (*a*) Boyd–Stille; (*b*) Thorek; (*c*) Stille–Matarasso.

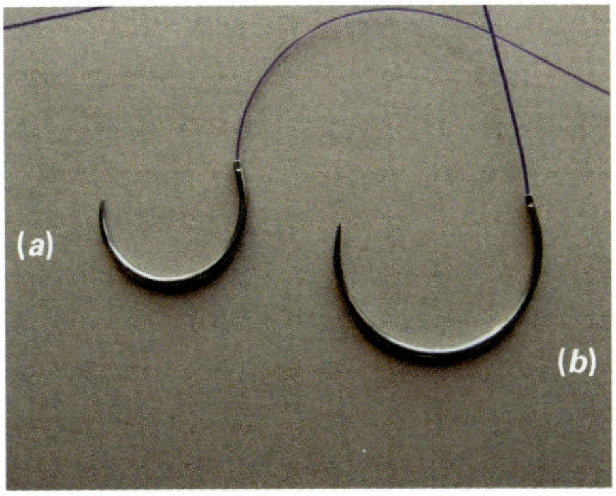

Figure 5.5 Our favourite needles for special situations: (*a*) 3-0 Monocryl on a 5/8-circle 26 mm round-bodied needle; (*b*) 2-0 Vicryl on a 5/8-circle 36 mm round-bodied needle. Both needles are very strong. (See Appendix A for suppliers.)

The choice of suture may be determined by what is available. Some stocks of chromic catgut are unreliable, and we prefer to avoid its use. Vicryl or Dexon, 0, 2/0 and 3/0, would be the first choice of most surgeons, if available. Newer monofilament absorbable sutures are very nice to use.

For closure of the bladder, half-circle, 26 mm, strong, round-bodied needles are best. For more advanced fistula work, eyed J-needles are a great help.

The perfect needle for a suture is a ready-mounted 5/8-circle 26 mm needle, but this is expensive. We reserve it for suturing in difficult corners and deep situations. Once you have used 5/8-circle needles, you will never want to use anything else!

A larger cutting needle is used for suturing vaginal mucosa.

Operating table

An operating table that tilts to at least 50° and has shoulder rests is advisable for the full range of surgery (Figure 5.6). Simpler fistula repairs can be carried out with a more modest tilt and without shoulder rests.

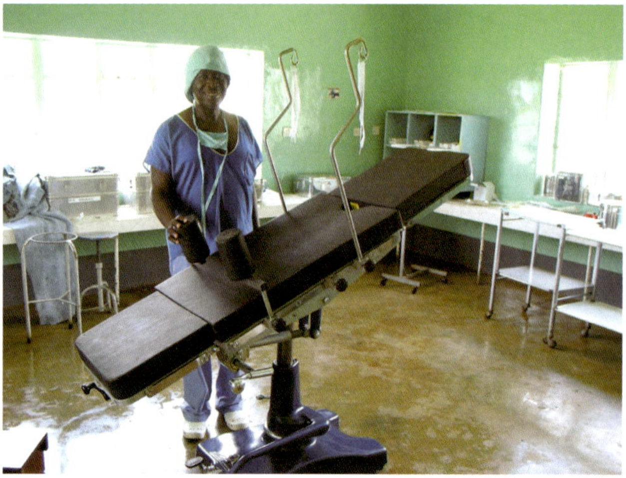

Figure 5.6 A tilting table.

Lighting

A simple spotlight is sufficient for easy cases (Figure 5.7). In situations where the electricity supply is erratic, it may be necessary to operate by daylight (Figure 5.8) – position the table close to a large window. On the other hand, in some hospitals, a full range of lighting equipment may be available (Figure 5.9).

As we operate in a variety of hospitals with unpredictable lighting (Figure 5.10), we prefer to have our own independent lighting source (Figure 5.11). The clip-on lamp can be used on one's own spectacles or supplied attached to a neutral spectacle frame. The rechargeable battery can be switched on and off through a sterile gown and provides brilliant spot illumination for 4 hours (see Appendix A for suppliers).

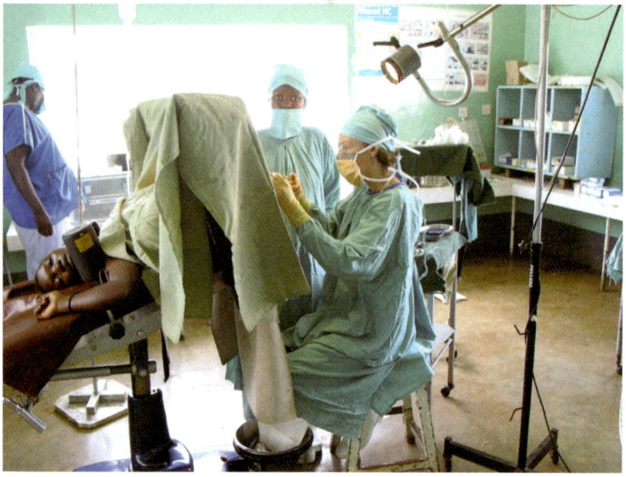

Figure 5.7 A simple spotlight.

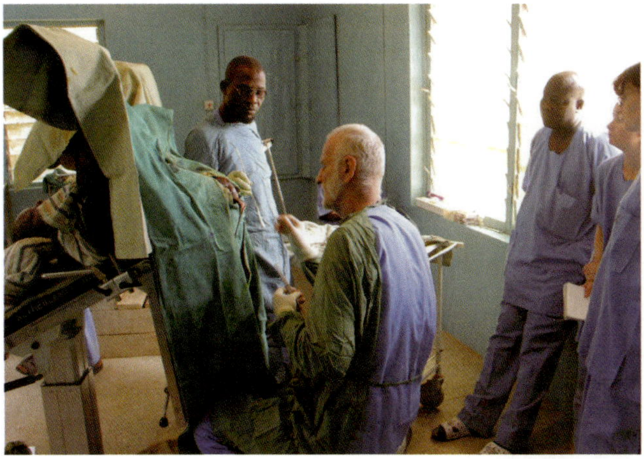

Figure 5.8 Kees Waaldijk operating by daylight in Katsina.

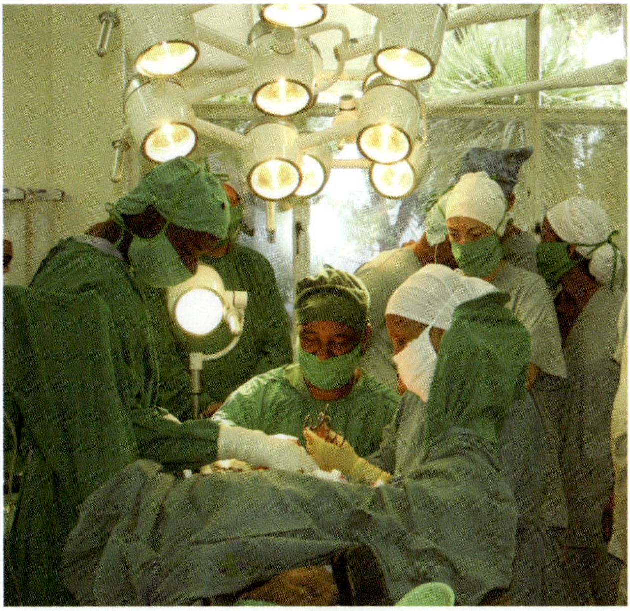

Figure 5.9 A sophisticated lighting set-up in the Addis Ababa Fistula Hospital.

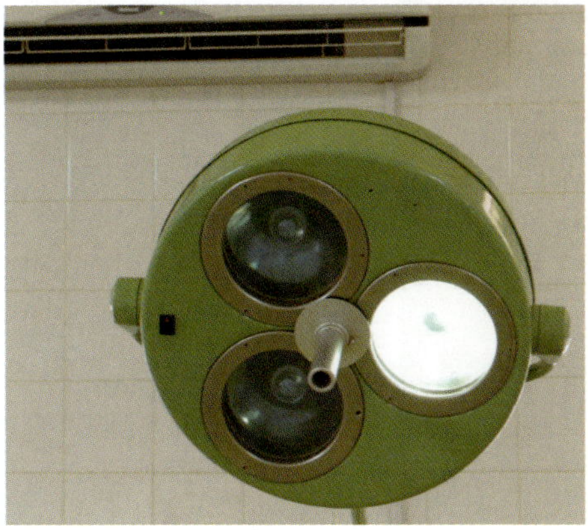

Figure 5.10 Faulty lighting equipment – a common situation in African hospitals.

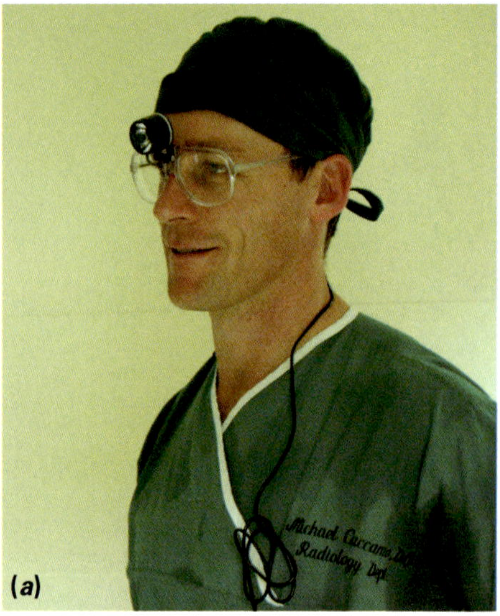

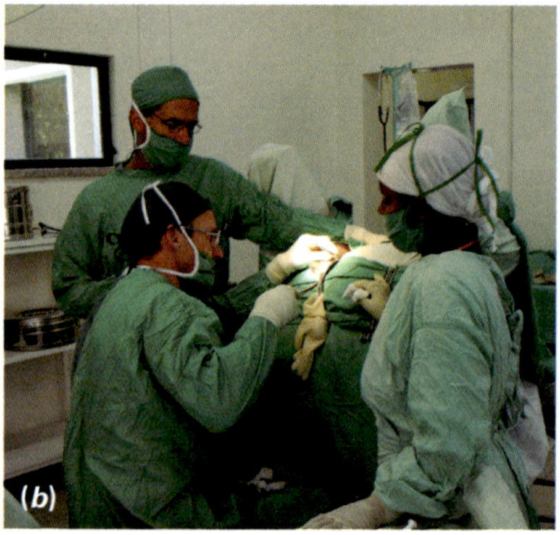

Figure 5.11 (*a*) Andrew Browning wearing a portable headlight. (*b*) Operating with the headlight.

Position on the table

The steeper the head-down position, the better (Figure 5.12). However, very high-quality shoulder rests are essential for this. If these are not available then it is important that the patient's buttocks be well over the end of the table and the thighs well flexed over the abdomen (Figure 5.13).

Surgeon's position

The surgeon should be in a comfortable position (Figures 5.15 and 5.16).

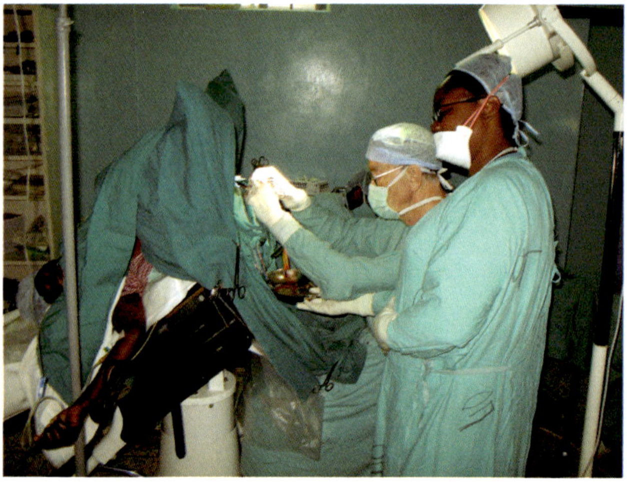

Figure 5.12 John Kelly demonstrating the correct head-down position of the patient.

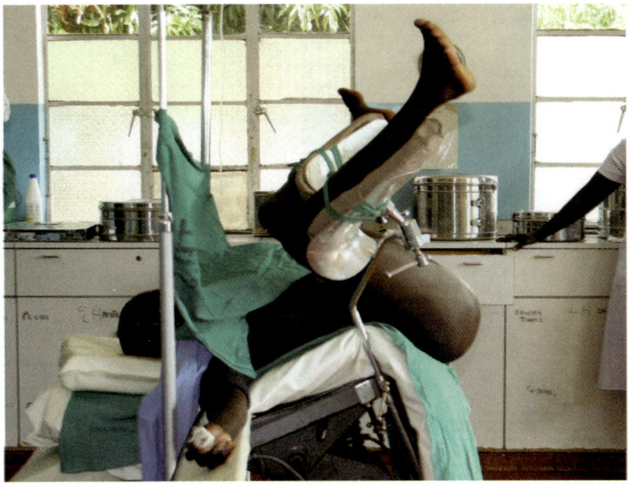

Figure 5.13 If there are no shoulder rests, the patient's buttocks must be well over the end of the table and the thighs well flexed over the abdomen to prevent her from slipping down.

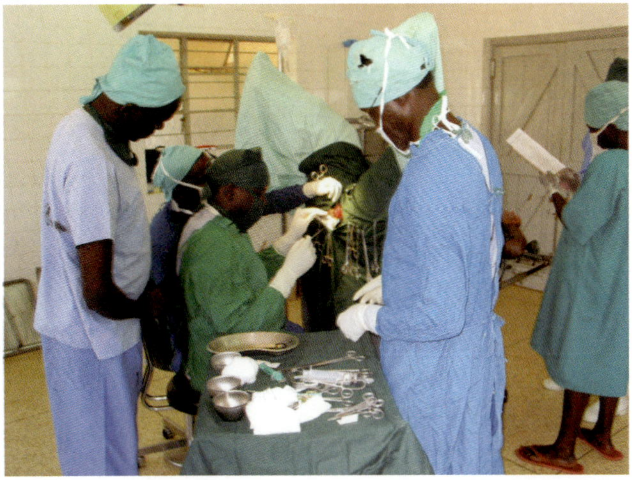

Figure 5.14 In this operating theatre, the old table will not tilt much, but the patient's buttocks are over the edge and her legs are supported high up out of the way, giving clear vision to the assistant and scrub nurse.

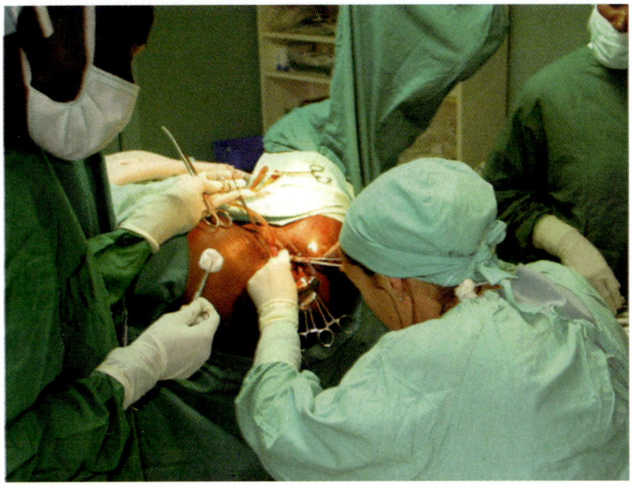

Figure 5.15 This surgeon is most uncomfortable – the table is too low.

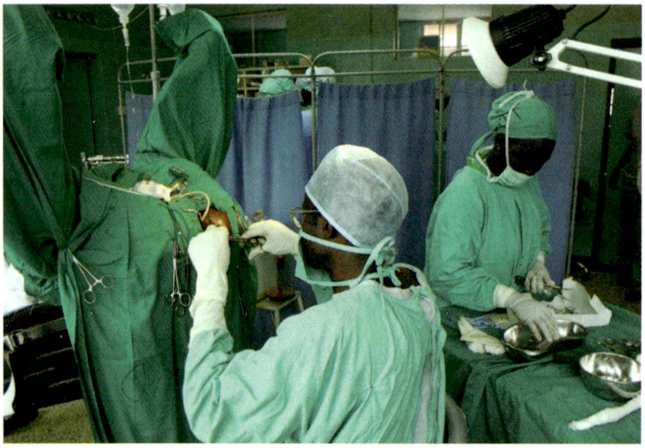

Figure 5.16 The operating field should be at eye level.

6 The Operations

BASIC PRINCIPLES

Basic principles are described here; strategies for specific situations are discussed in later sections. The basic principles in the repair of a fistula are:

- adequate exposure
- protection of the ureters
- separation of the vagina from the bladder around the fistula
- mobilization of enough bladder after excision of scar to allow a tension-free closure of the defect that shows no leakage on dye test
- support for the urethra when it is deficient.

These principles are now described and illustrated.

Fistulae come in all different shapes, sizes and sites, but the basic principles of the surgical technique can be applied to all. Distal (the urethral end) and proximal are used to denote the parts of the fistula in the operative descriptions (Figure 6.1).

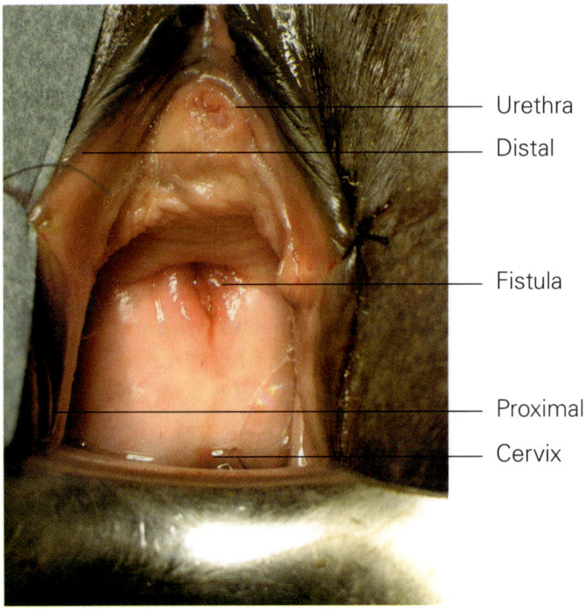

Figure 6.1 Definition of 'distal' and 'proximal'.

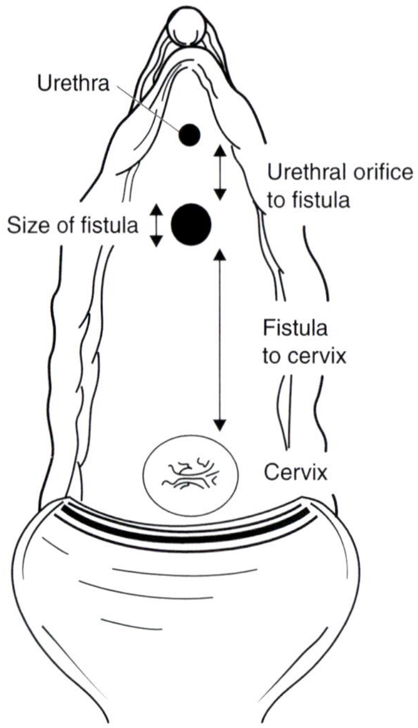

Figure 6.2 Measurements to make.

Documentation of the fistula

The fistula must be described. We use Goh's classification (see Chapter 1).

First, the vagina is assessed for depth and stenosis. The fistula is described by its site, size and surrounding scar. By palpation, an attempt should be made to determine whether the bladder has been separated from the urethra. The cervix should be inspected and palpated for damage, and the posterior wall checked for any missed rectal injury.

An attempt should be made to measure the distance from the external urethral orifice to the distal fistula margin (Figure 6.2) and to estimate the size of the bladder (Figure 6.3). (A sound or metal catheter marked in centimetres is ideal, although a practical alternative is to know the length of one's thumb's distal phalanx for estimating urethral length.)

It is vital to tap the interior of the bladder to detect stones (Figure 6.3). *To overlook a stone during a repair is a disaster.* Any stones should be recognized and removed before the repair. Although calculi occurred in only 3% of our Ugandan series, most were in fact easily detected before the patient reached theatre (see 'Bladder stones' later in this chapter).

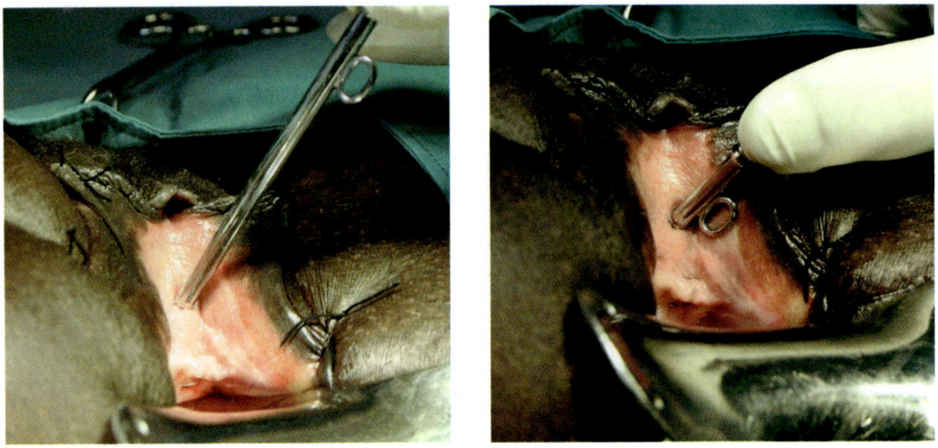

Figure 6.3 Sounding the bladder for stones and size.

Access

The labia are first sutured laterally to improve access, and a swab is sutured to cover the anus (Figure 6.4).

In more complex cases, it is common to find scarring inside the vagina that is sufficiently severe to prevent the insertion of the Auvard speculum. Most commonly, there is a thick band of scar on the posterior vaginal wall. The scar is released by incising the band laterally either side, staying away from the rectum and the bladder. If there is any doubt, a finger can be inserted into the rectum for guidance. Incising the scar in this way may result in a reasonable vaginal capacity. In cases of extensive scarring, the lateral incisions can be brought infero-laterally out into the ischio-rectal fossa, making large episiotomies. An Auvard speculum can then be introduced, exposing the fistula.

More frequently, a simple episiotomy, bilateral on occasions, will improve access greatly (Figure 6.5). Beginners will need to make episiotomies more frequently than experienced surgeons.

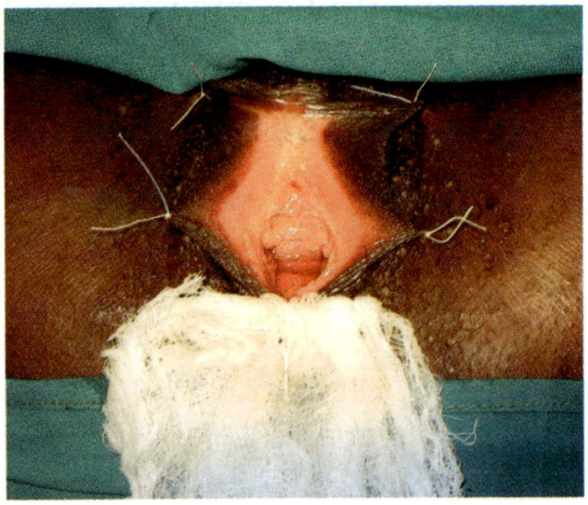

Figure 6.4 The labia are sutured and the anus is covered.

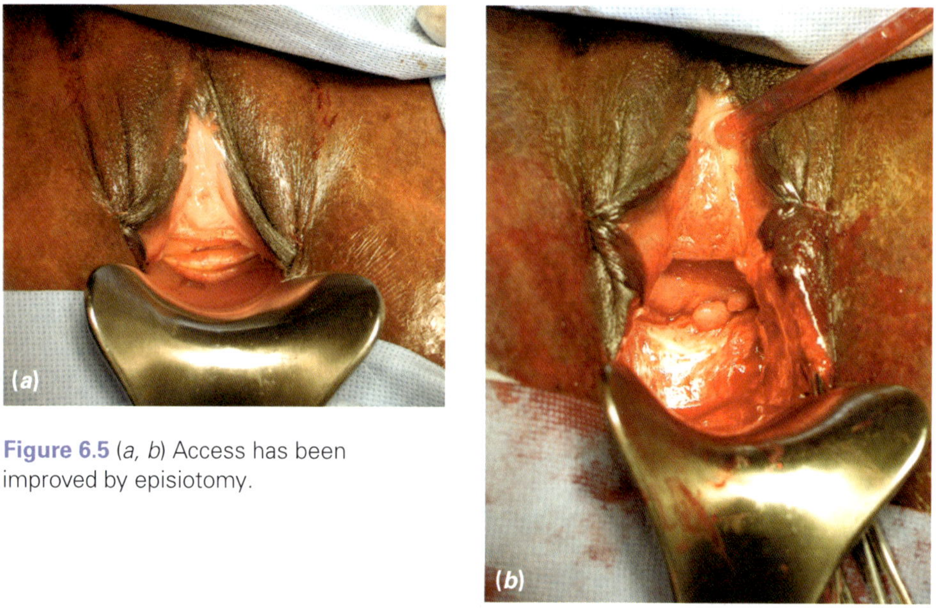

Figure 6.5 (*a, b*) Access has been improved by episiotomy.

Some surgeons infiltrate the vaginal wall around the fistula margin with a mild haemostatic agent (1:200 000 adrenaline (epinephrine)). This reduces blood loss, thus aiding dissection. There is a small risk of reactionary haemorrhage when the effect wears off. Others prefer isotonic saline. If the infiltrate is being introduced into the correct tissue plane beneath the vaginal skin, it should be introduced easily (except when there is severe scarring). Although many surgeons do not infiltrate at all, we believe that it is helpful for beginners.

Initially, the vaginal wall distal to the fistula should be held with the Allis forceps. Upward traction brings the fistula into view (Figure 6.6).

The proximal margin of the fistula is incised, with the incision being made through the full thickness of the vaginal wall, but not into the bladder. The incision is

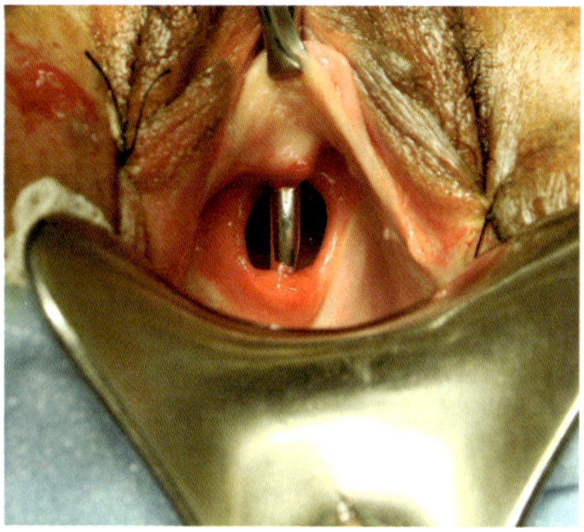

Figure 6.6 The fistula is brought into view by upward traction.

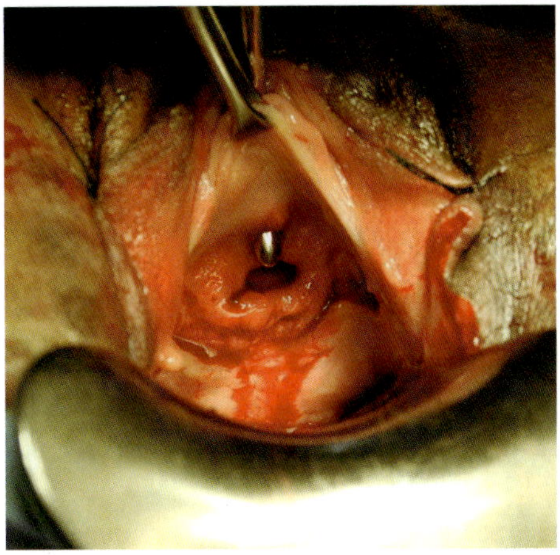

Figure 6.7 Access for dissection is facilitated by advancing the incision onto the lateral walls of the vagina.

advanced onto the lateral walls of the vagina from the left and right angles of the fistula. This assists with access for the dissection (Figure 6.7). A size 15 blade is most suitable for this step.

The proximal bladder wall is grasped with the Allis forceps and held by the assistant. The surgeon holds the vaginal wall with dissecting forceps and gently applies counter-traction to expose the operative plane. A combination of sharp and blunt dissection (Figure 6.8) is used to develop the plane between the bladder and the vagina. Note that the bladder and vagina are held apart with the Allis forceps to show the space between them. Opening the tips of scissors in this plane helps to develop it. Tension should be maintained on both the bladder and vaginal walls during dissection. It is important to stay just under the vagina. Bleeding is a warning that the bladder wall has been entered.

The dissection is extended laterally until the angles of the fistula are free. The dissection can appear rather extensive to the novice fistula surgeon, but it must be

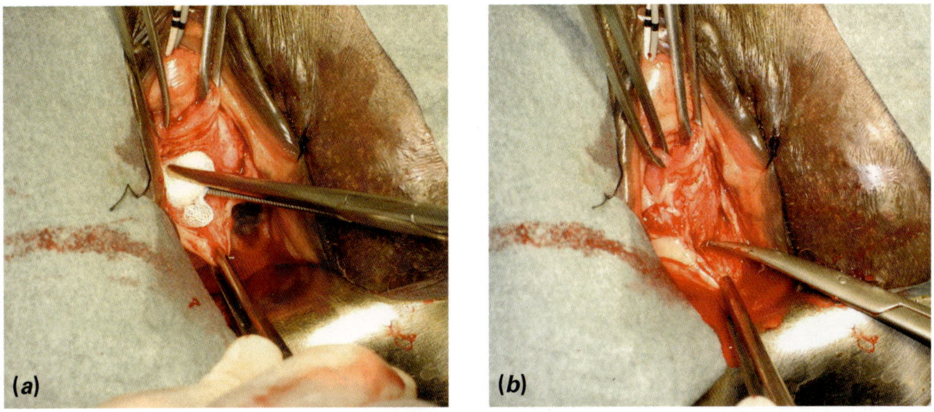

Figure 6.8 (*a, b*) The plane between the bladder and vagina is developed using a combination of sharp and blunt dissection.

extensive enough to free the bladder off the vagina to enable a completely tension-free closure of the bladder. Much more dissection will be done in a proximal direction, up to or beyond the cervix, than over the urethra, which is fixed. *This is the most crucial lesson for the fistula surgeon. If the bladder is closed under any tension, the operation will fail.*

In more severe injuries, the lateral margin of the fistula is the pubic bone, and clearly a different strategy is required. Management of this situation is discussed in 'Circumferential fistulae' later in this chapter.

Protection of ureters

It is wise to identify the ureters in all cases except for the very smallest fistulae. The ureters enter the bladder just distal to the level of the cervix and are indentified with a ureteric probe (Figure 6.9). (If the ureters are difficult to identify, 20 mg intravenous furosemide and a bolus of intravenous fluid will produce an intermittent spurt of urine from each ureteric orifice, aiding localization.) If the ureters are close to the fistula margin, they should be catheterized, advancing the catheters up to the renal pelvis and then withdrawing them slightly. This is done to avoid incorporating the ureters in the repair (even so, ureters have been injured during dissection – see Chapter 13). The catheters are brought out through the urethra by either threading them into a metal catheter or pulling them through with a small curved artery forceps (Figure 6.10). They are then secured onto the mons pubis with a simple stitch. Wherever possible, it is best to catheterize the ureters before beginning dissection.

After the proximal margin has been mobilized sufficiently, attention is given to the distal margin. Most surgeons new to fistula surgery find this plane difficult to dissect, especially when the fistula is pulled up behind the symphysis.

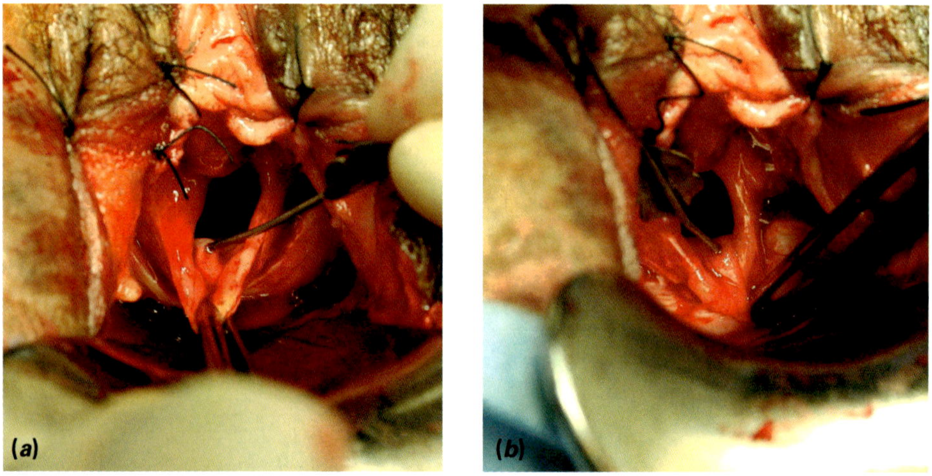

Figure 6.9 (*a*) Right ureteric orifice identified. (*b*) Left ureteric orifice identified.

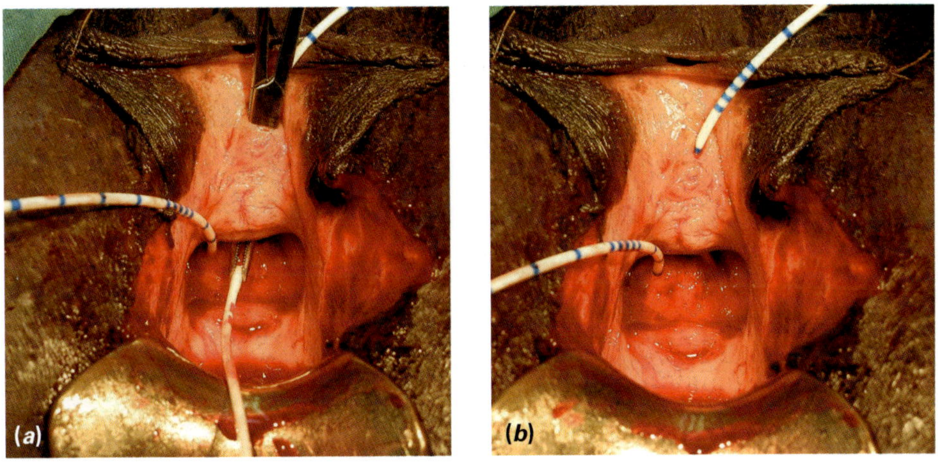

Figure 6.10 (*a, b*) Ureteric catheters are pulled through the urethra. In a case like this, they would be removed at the end of the operation.

The metal catheter is a useful retractor in the urethra, and it also helps the surgeon to gauge the thickness of the tissue planes, which are thin when approaching the urethra. To help with this, a small vertical incision may be made from the upper margin of the fistula distally in the midline. The incision around the distal fistula margin joins the previous proximal dissection. A lateral extension is made down the axis of the vagina. This may have already been done from the lateral ends of the proximal dissection. This is particularly important when a fistula is pulled up behind the symphysis.

The distal flap must now be dissected off the proximal urethra and para-urethral region. The elevation of the distal flap should always commence with dissection at its lateral edge (Figure 6.11), working towards the midline and repeating the same step on the other side. If this is not done, the urethra can easily be damaged and the flap torn. If the fistula is pulled up behind the symphysis, the right-angled tips of the Thorek scissors (see Chapter 5) are most helpful. The Allis forceps are again useful in providing traction to bring the upper margin into view and in providing traction and counter-traction to find the correct tissue plane.

When the surgeon judges that there has been enough dissection to enable a tension-free closure, the reflected tissue is sewn to the labia on each side with a suture (Figure 6.12).

The fistula edge is trimmed of any scar tissue or residual vaginal skin. The angles are examined again to ensure that they are not tethered to the inferior pubic ramus on either side. If so, further dissection is needed.

The fistula is then repaired with interrupted 00 absorbable sutures. The vagina is a confined area in which to operate, and suturing can pose a problem. Small, strong needles are needed. Fish-hook (J) needles or 5/8-circle needles are ideal. The angles are secured first, taking bites distal, proximal and lateral to the fistula angle. The

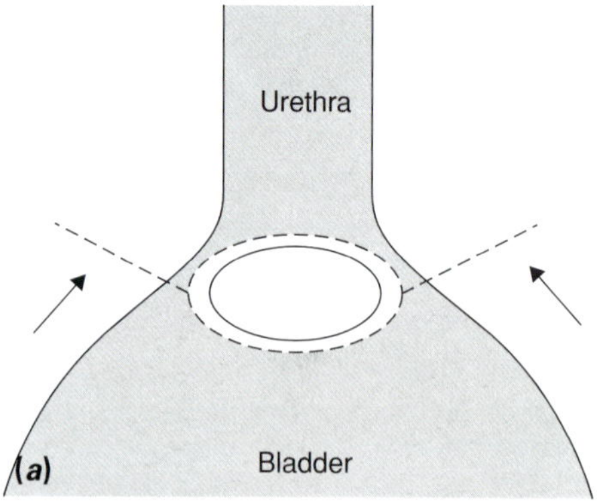

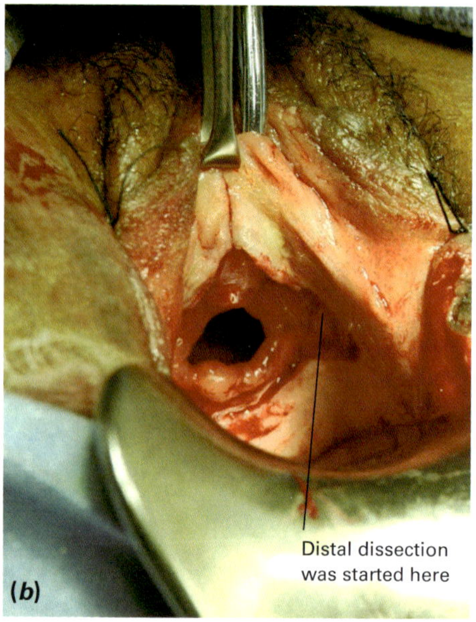

Figure 6.11 (*a*) To elevate the distal flap, the dissection is always started laterally, working towards the urethra from both sides. (*b*) Distal dissection. Note that a small vertical incision has been made though the vaginal skin over the urethra. This is optional.

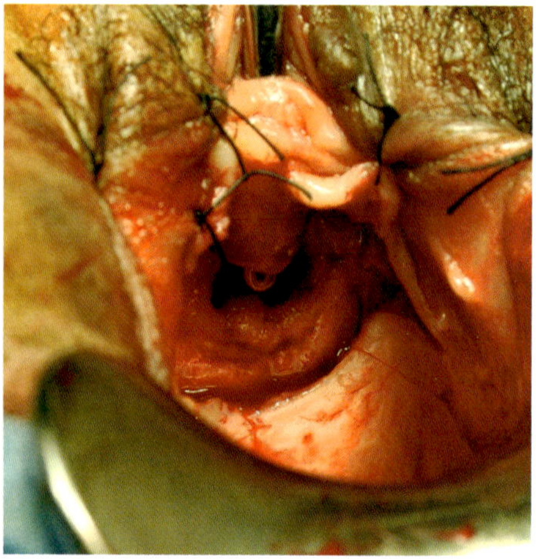

Figure 6.12 The distal flaps have been sutured up out of the way. The extent of dissection can be seen. Note the metal catheter in the urethra.

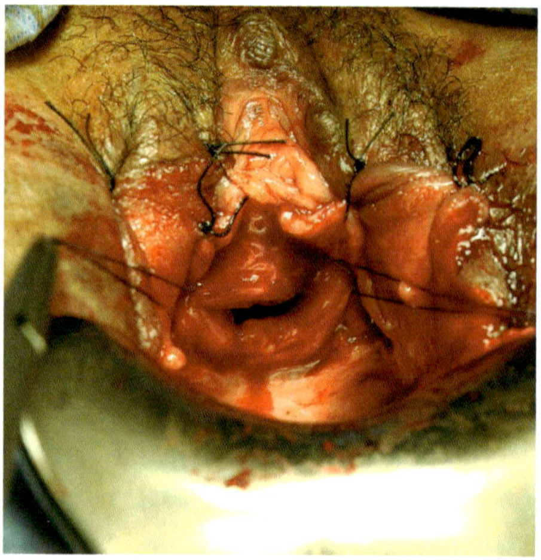

Figure 6.13 The two corner sutures have been inserted and held.

corner sutures are clipped after tying for identification (Figure 6.13). For the central sutures, it may be easier if they are not tied until all have been inserted.

It is very important to ensure that there is no protrusion of bladder mucosa at any point along the suture line. This is especially so at the corners. The suture includes only the bladder muscle; the mucosa is excluded from the repair so as to invert it into the bladder (Figure 6.14).

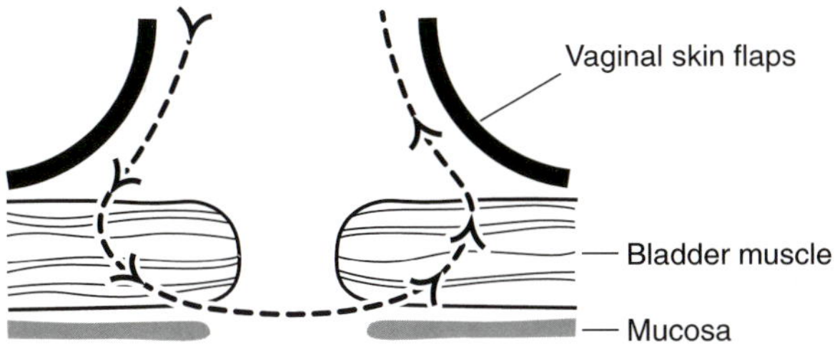

Figure 6.14 The suture includes only the bladder muscle, avoiding the mucosa.

One layer or two?

Traditionally, two layers have been recommended, but there are many surgeons (including ourselves) who use only one layer as a general rule. The bites must be accurately and evenly spaced. One technical tip is never to try to hold forceps and needle holder while tying knots. It is much easier to judge tension accurately when both hands are free (Figure 6.15). A second layer should never be used when suturing to proximal urethra. There is a high chance that this would cut out or effectively shorten the urethra. However, in other situations when there is available tissue, we do recommend that beginners add a second layer.

Once the repair has been completed (Figure 6.16), a dye test is performed to ensure sound closure of the bladder (Figure 6.17). A no. 16 Foley catheter is passed, saline coloured with methylene blue is introduced into the bladder (around 100 cm^3 should suffice) and the suture line is checked for leaks. A common error is to use the dye too concentrated. Leakage from the repair or urethra will stain everything too much, making identification of the leak difficult.

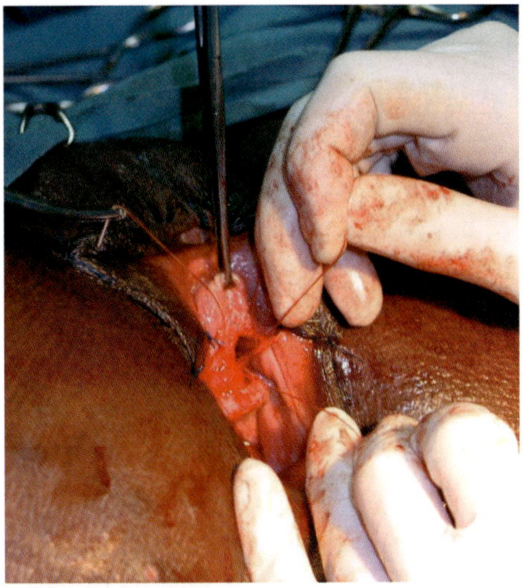

Figure 6.15 Both hands should be free of instruments while tying knots.

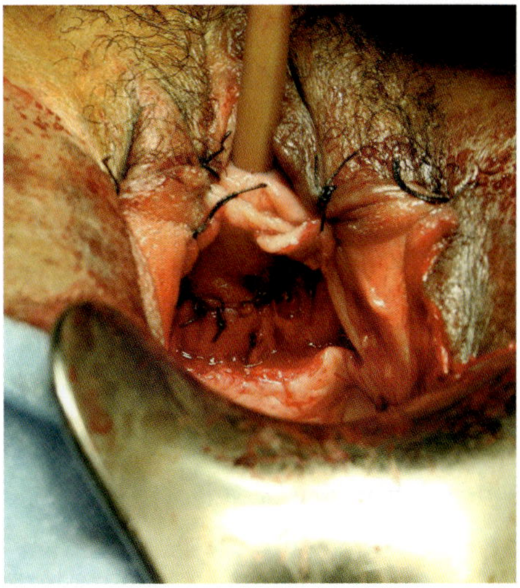

Figure 6.16 Completed repair.

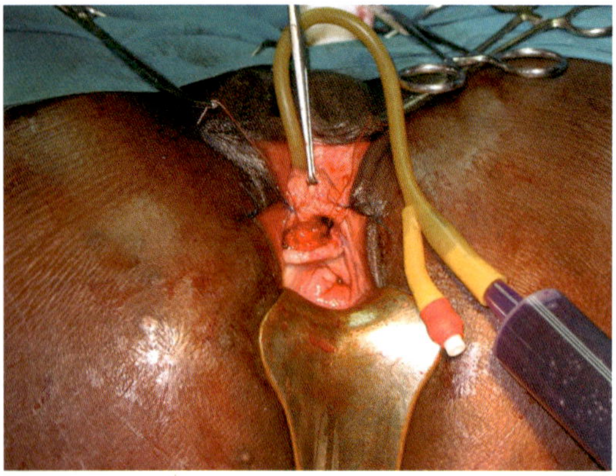

Figure 6.17 A dye test in progress.

A more objective method is to fill the bladder via a filter funnel or open syringe, pouring in the dye until the intravesical pressure is about 30 cmH_2O. This is judged by the height of the fluid in the vertically held catheter. The volume instilled gives a measure of the functional capacity of the bladder.

A patient may have more than one fistula, so it is important to inspect the rest of the vagina carefully for leaks. It may be necessary to gently press on the urethral meatus with a swab to prevent dye leaking out of the urethra and spilling into the vagina, making interpretation of the test difficult. If the dye test is satisfactory, pressure over the urethra can be released to look for a urethral leak. Whether this predicts stress incontinence remains to be determined.

Sometimes, an additional suture is required, but, if the leak is not controlled by one or two additional sutures, it is better to take at least part of the repair down and begin again rather than inserting more and more sutures that will only strangle tissue.

Vaginal closure

This is performed with interrupted sutures (Figure 6.18). It is usual to close the vagina completely where possible, but, if there has been a more extensive dissection or there is marked loss of vaginal tissue, it is may be better to leave some gaps. If the vaginal incision is closed tightly after a large dissection, an infected haematoma could burst into the bladder and/or the vagina, whereas, if the vagina is partly open, blood or infection can readily drain out.

Haemostasis

Actively bleeding vessels should always be secured by an under-running suture, but sometimes a degree of continuous oozing has to be accepted. This may be reduced by greater head-down tilt or dilute adrenaline-soaked swabs, and finally controlled by packing.

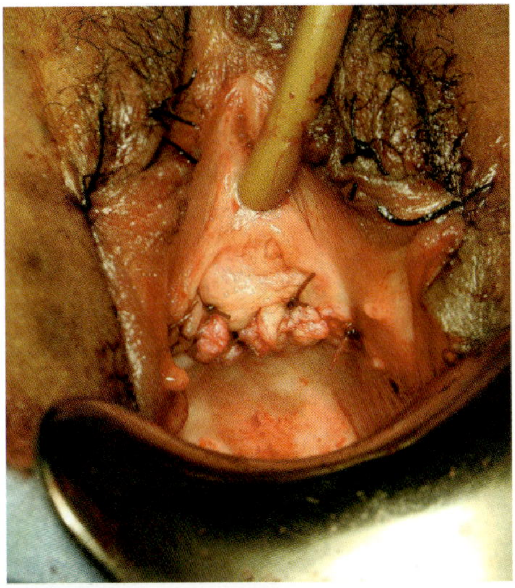

Figure 6.18 The vaginal skin has been closed with a mattress suture.

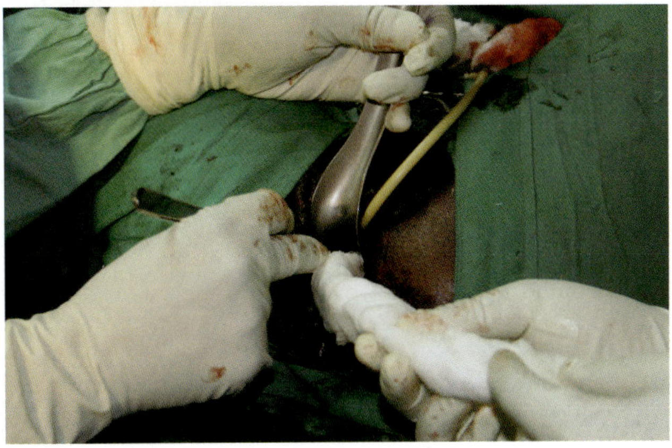

Figure 6.19 The repair should be protected with a Sims speculum when inserting the pack.

Vaginal packing

It is traditional to finish by packing the vagina with gauze soaked in antiseptic solution. However, this may not be necessary. Residual venous oozing is common at the end of large cases, and a firm pack may stop this. It is important to realize, however, that a pack may prevent the recognition of serious bleeding for several hours. There is probably no need to pack in most simple dry cases, but, to simplify nursing, it is better to have an 'all-or-none' policy, as a retained pack is a disaster. We still prefer a pack for all cases, with its removal the next day.

When packing, the site of the repair should always be protected with a Sims speculum (Figure 6.19).

Securing the indwelling catheter

Some surgeons prefer to suture the indwelling catheter onto the labia whereas others just tape the catheter (see Chapter 11). The aim is to ensure that the balloon of the catheter does not put pressure on the repair site. This should not be a problem for high vaginal fistulae, where the repair site is away from the bladder neck, but, for those fistulae involving the urethra or bladder neck, we prefer to suture the catheter in place to prevent any pressure or traction on the repair. The important thing to remember is to keep the bladder empty with the catheter draining well during the 2 weeks after the operation.

The next section describes the selection of cases for a beginner, with the more challenging fistulae being described in subsequent sections.

SELECTION OF CASES FOR THE BEGINNER

We shall repeatedly emphasize that selection of cases is the most important aspect of fistula management that a trainee must learn.

It must be remembered that to attempt a case beyond one's capabilities is not only demoralizing for the surgeon but a disaster for the patient, as the best chance of cure is always the first operation.

Of all the new cases presenting, only about one-quarter will be suitable for a beginner. History taking does not help that much in selecting the easy ones. A small hole leaks just as much as a big one.

There are some clues that should make one suspicious of a serious or difficult fistula:

- Neurological weakness (usually foot drop), even if it has recovered, suggests a difficult case.
- Rectal fistulae usually occur in association with a serious bladder injury. This does not apply to anal sphincter injuries, which often occur in isolation.
- Fistulae following caesarean section are often in the region of the cervix and therefore high.
- A fistula following hysterectomy for a ruptured uterus will usually be in the vault or be due to an accidental ureteric injury.

The only clue to a potentially easy case is when a patient gives a history of pregnancies in spite of having a fistula. Clearly, there cannot have been too much damage to the genital tract. About 10% of our cases have had pregnancies while suffering from a fistula.

Examination is the key to selection. The features to look for are:

- a vagina without shortening or stenosis
- a fistula that is easily palpable or visible, and that is small, soft and accessible, but not too close to the cervix or to the external urethral orifice.

There is no need to examine such a patient under anaesthesia. If the fistula cannot be easily seen in the conscious patient using a Sims speculum then it is not a simple case.

In summary, novice surgeons should confine themselves to:

- small fistulae not involving the urethra
- those with minimal scar
- those that are easily accessible.

An ideal case

Unfortunately, only 10% of cases are as easy as the one shown in Figure 6.20.

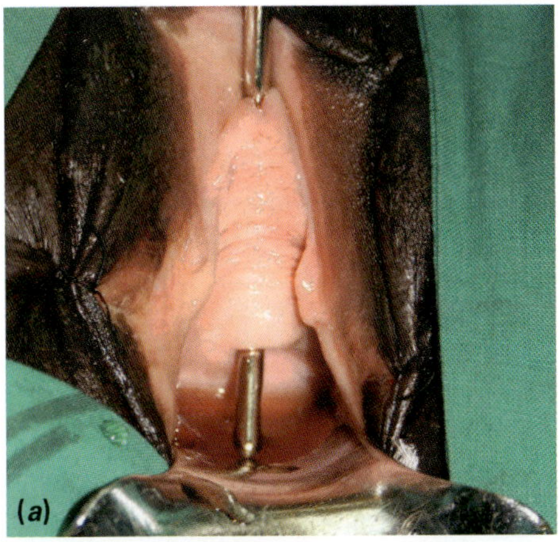
(*a*)

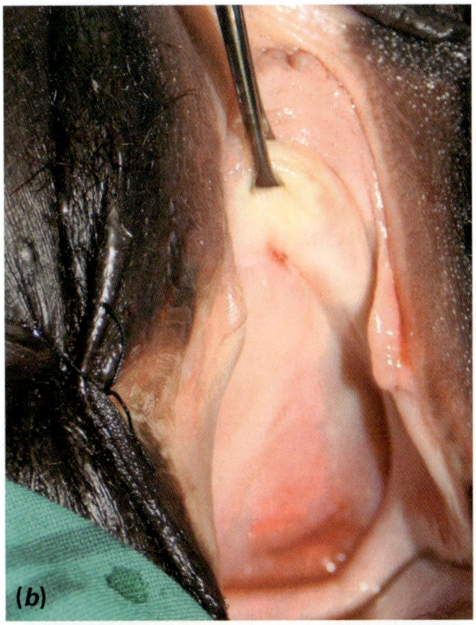
(*b*)

Figure 6.20 (*a*) A small mid-vaginal fistula (Goh's type 1al). (*b*) The distal wall of the vagina is held up with Allis forceps to expose the fistula. It is seen well distal to the cervix.

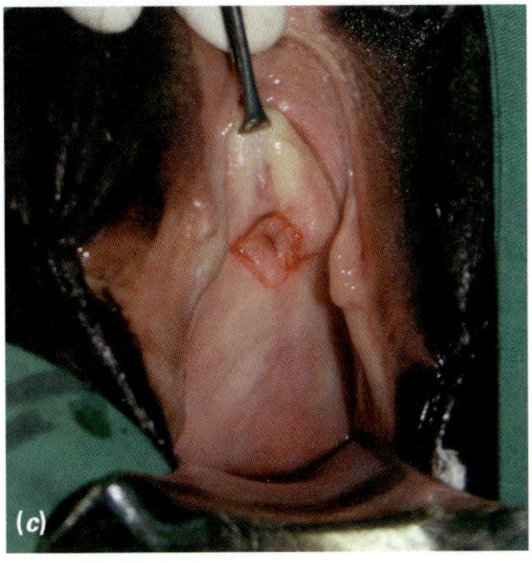
(*c*)

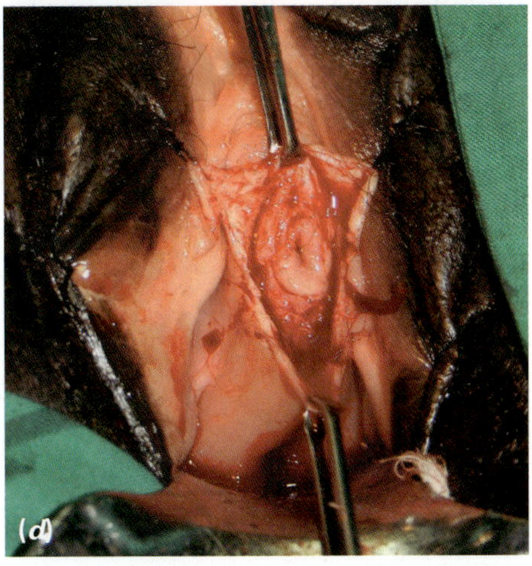
(*d*)

(*c*) Incision around the fistula. (*d*) Extent of mobilization. The bladder margin will be trimmed of vaginal mucosa and inverted with one layer of sutures, taking good bites of bladder proximal and distal to the defect. *(continued)*

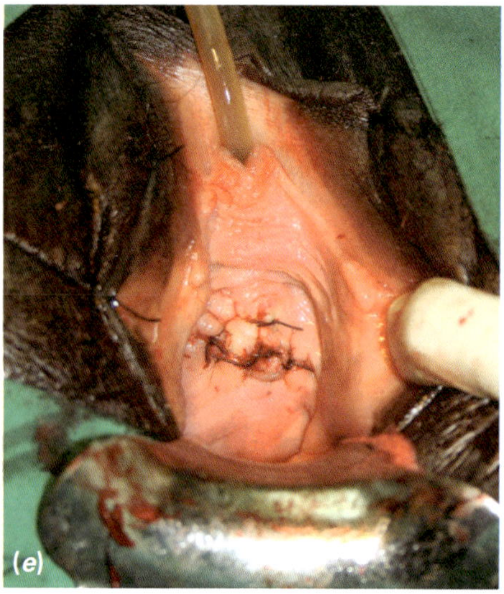

Figure 6.20 (*e*) The vagina is closed over the repaired bladder.

Some relatively easy cases

Some other examples of cases suitable for a trainee are shown in Figures 6.21–6.25.

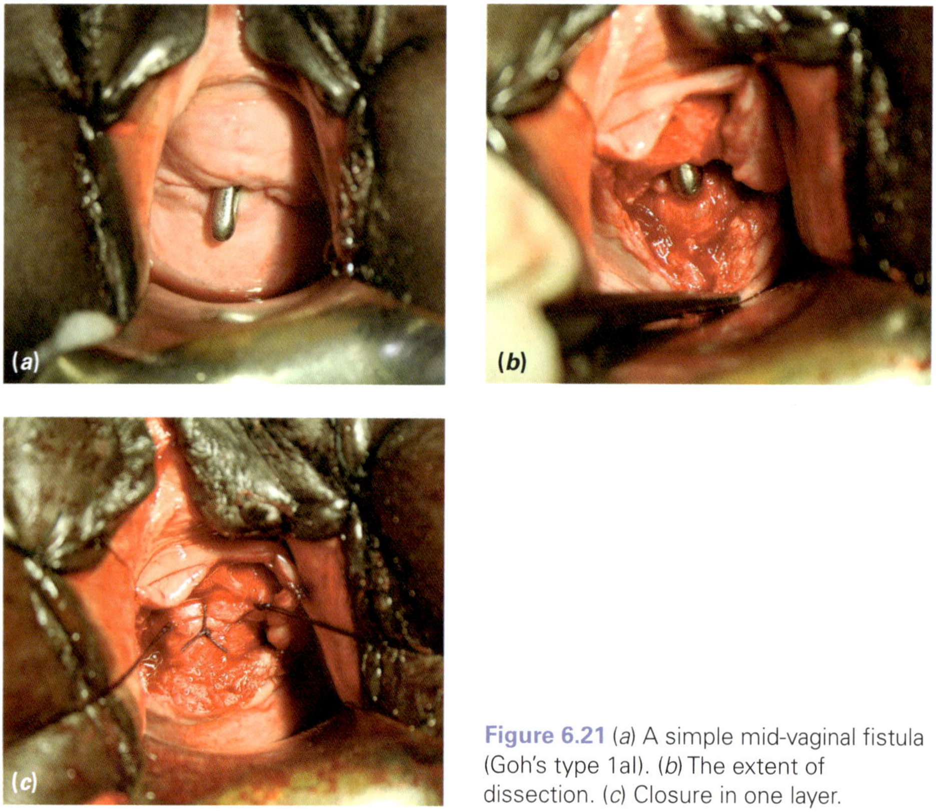

Figure 6.21 (*a*) A simple mid-vaginal fistula (Goh's type 1al). (*b*) The extent of dissection. (*c*) Closure in one layer.

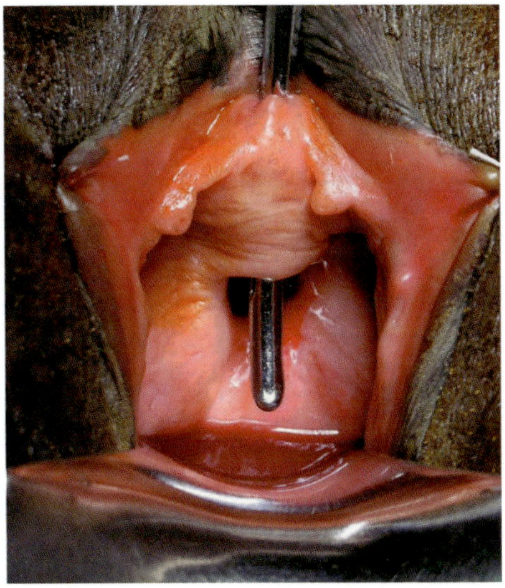

Figure 6.22 A medium-size fistula at the junction of the urethra and bladder. The margins of the fistula are soft and are clearly seen. The urethra is just intact (Goh's type 2bI).

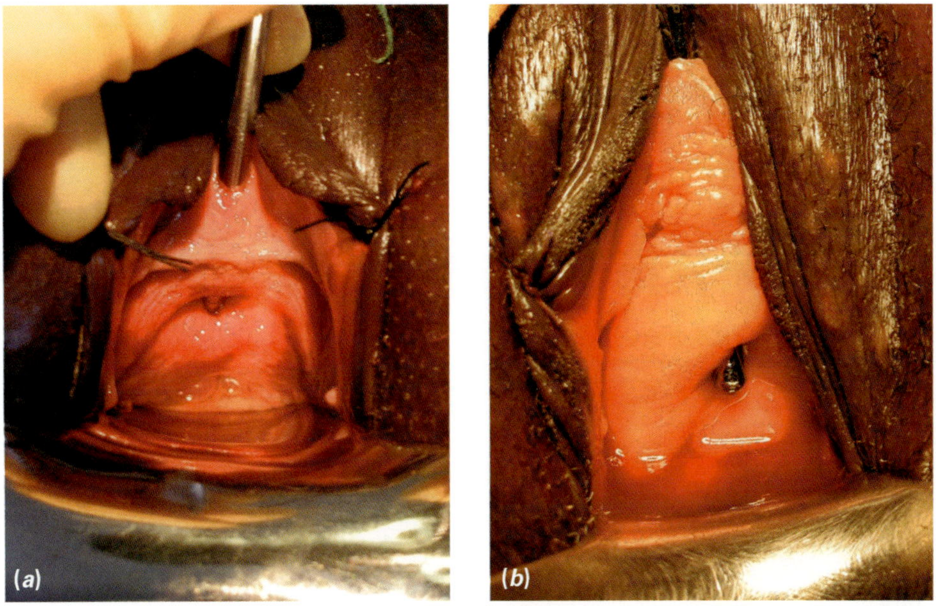

Figure 6.23 Two simple fistulae. Note that the fistula in (*a*) is not as accessible as that in (*b*). The former will become much easier after an episiotomy.

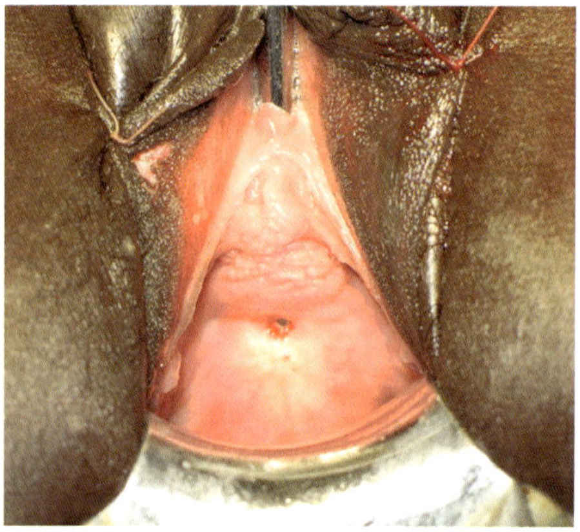

Figure 6.24 The hole in this case appears tiny, but there is considerable fibrosis around it. The scar tissue must be excised, so a generous mobilization will be required to reach healthy bladder.

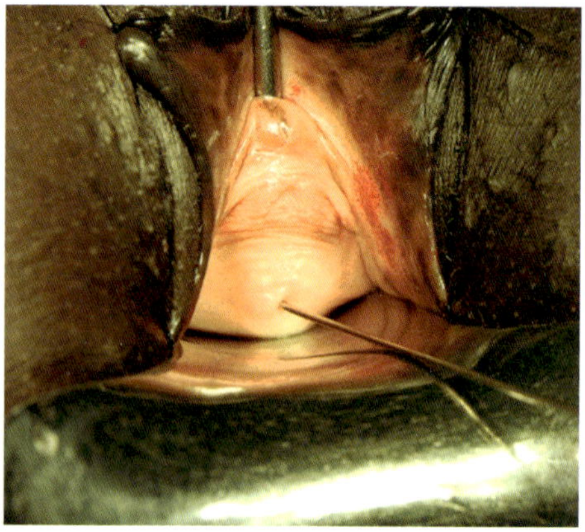

Figure 6.25 This pinhole fistula is easy to see, but can be quite troublesome to close. The probe should be kept in the fistula during the dissection, otherwise the track may be lost.

Some difficult cases

The cases shown in Figures 6.26–6.29 are more difficult, and should not be attempted by a beginner.

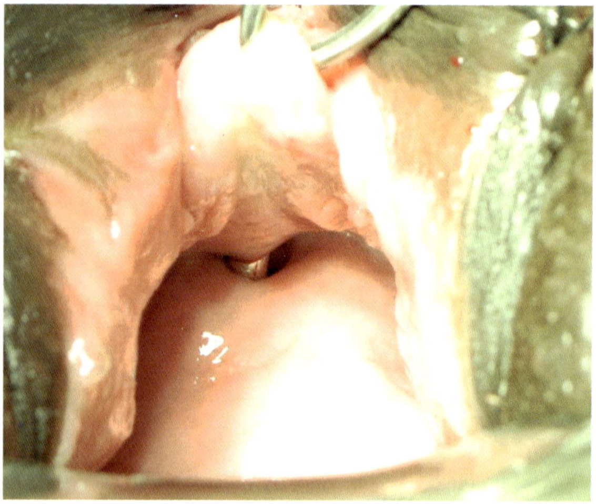

Figure 6.26 This juxta-urethral fistula is pulled up behind the symphysis, making access difficult. There is also almost complete separation of urethra and bladder (Goh's type 2aIII).

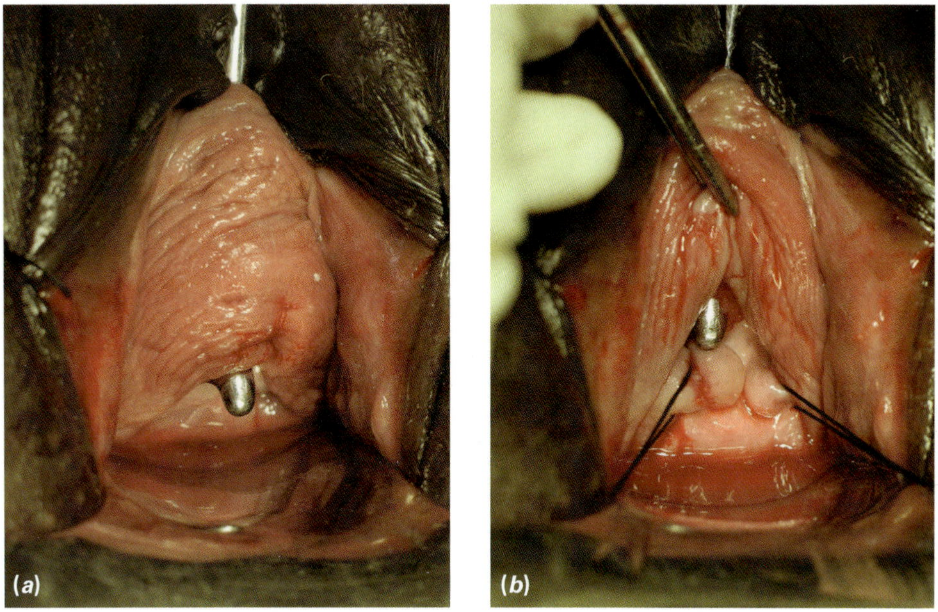

Figure 6.27 (*a, b*) This juxta-cervical fistula opens high into an open cervical canal. It is a challenging case to repair, but has an excellent prognosis because the urethro-vesical junction is undamaged.

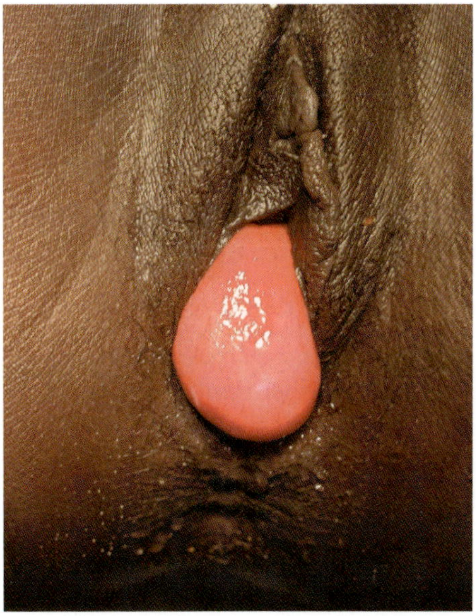

Figure 6.28 The defect in the vagina here is so large that the bladder has prolapsed, but this is perfectly curable by a regular fistula surgeon.

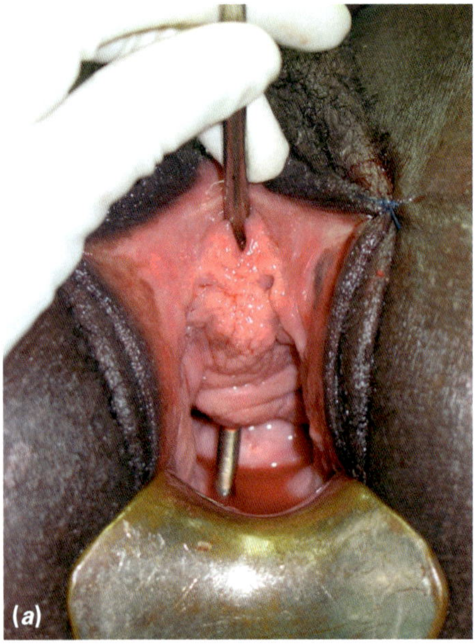

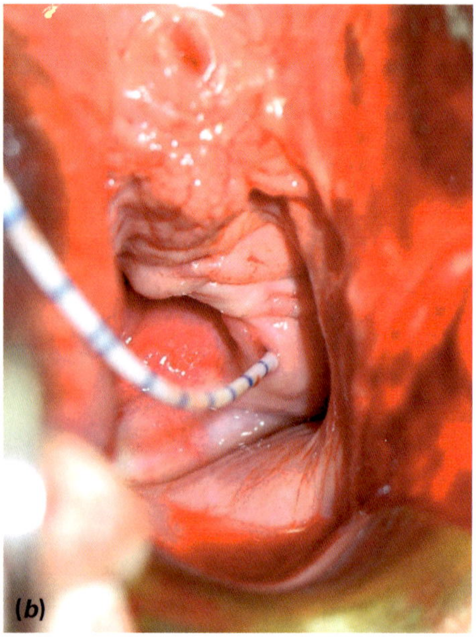

Figure 6.29 (*a,b*) This is a large fistula high in the vagina and involving the cervix (Goh's type 1cIII). When fully exposed after an episiotomy, the ureteric orifice is seen on the edge of the fistula. This would be quite easy for an expert, but a novice could get into difficulty.

JUXTA-URETHRAL AND CIRCUMFERENTIAL FISTULAE

The following are discussed in this section:

- Management of juxta-urethral and circumferential fistulae
- Management of ureteric involvement.

The key to repair of the more complex fistulae is to understand the circumferential fistula.

Anyone reading standard textbook accounts of vesico-vaginal fistula repair may get the impression that the fistula is simply a hole in the base of the bladder that needs to be closed transversely in one or two layers. The concept of circumferential loss and the strategies for dealing with this are often glossed over.

In the majority of cases, the ischaemic injury occurs at the urethro-vesical junction. When there is complete separation of urethra and bladder, the defect is called circumferential. If the urethra and bladder are still together to some extent, the defect is, by tradition, called juxta-urethral.

The degrees of circumferential loss are illustrated in Figure 6.30. It must be appreciated that in the larger defects the antero-lateral bladder wall is adherent to the pubic rami. The practical point is to make the distinction between fistulae with a

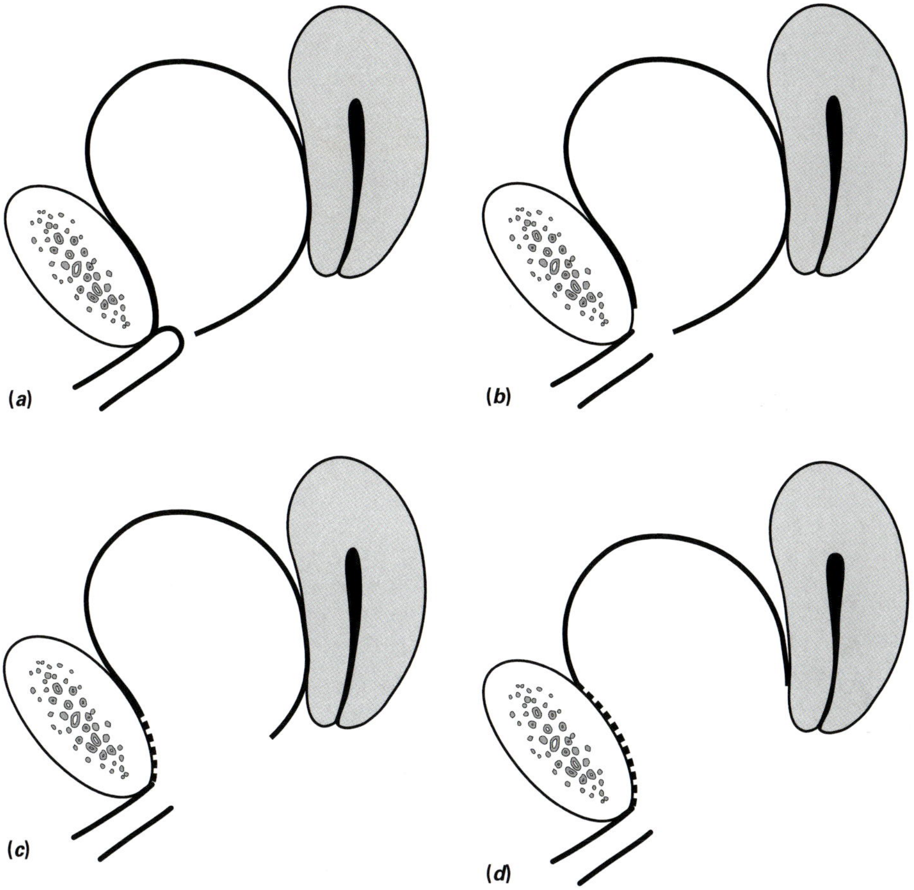

Figure 6.30 Degrees of circumferential tissue loss: (*a*) stenosed proximal urethra but negligible separation; (*b*) complete separation with a small gap; (*c*) more separation with pubic bone exposed – most of the anterior vaginal wall is missing; (*d*) major separation with significant loss of bladder volume.

small or negligible gap and those with a significant gap, as the management is different. In juxta-urethral fistulae, there is no complete separation. The defect extends around just part of the circumference of the bladder neck region and appears as a simple hole on inspection. The varying degrees of loss are shown in Figure 6.31.

There are two important things to consider:

- To what extent is there circumferential tissue loss (i.e. separation of bladder and urethra)?
- How much urethra has been destroyed?

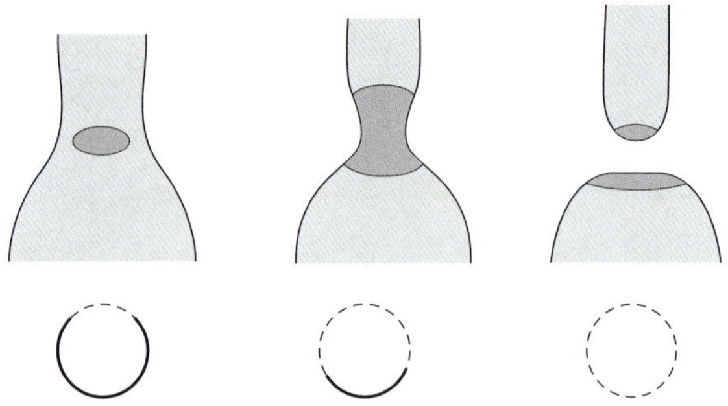

Figure 6.31 Degrees of incomplete detachment: (*a*) one-quarter loss; (*b*) three-quarters loss; (*c*) complete detachment. In the bottom row, the heavy shading indicates the muscle and mucosa remaining.

Extent of circumferential tissue loss

Is the circumferential tissue loss partial or complete? Many partial defects extend only around the superficial one-quarter and are easily closed by transverse sutures. In other cases, the defect extends around the sides, and the continuity between urethra and bladder is maintained on the deep aspect, where it is lightly adherent to the undersurface of the pubic arch. Here a three-quarters to one-half circle anastomosis of bladder to urethra is required. There will usually be no major discrepancy in size between urethra and bladder neck.

Where there is complete separation, a gap will be felt and seen. A circumferential re-anastomosis is generally recommended.

Extent of urethral destruction

The normal urethra is about 3.5 cm long. The urethra is almost always damaged to some extent in the cases under discussion. There is frequently a block in the proximal urethra, which needs to be dilated. The status of the urethra is best recorded by measuring or estimating the distance from the external urethral orifice to the distal fistula margin (it is helpful to know the length of one's own distal phalanx and length from nail tip to nail bed. Goh's classification from 1 to 4 may then be applied. Urethral length is the major prognostic factor for stress incontinence. When the urethra is short, we recommend a urethral support procedure that is described later in this chapter.

Operative steps for non-circumferential fistulae

A non-circumferential fistula in the region of the bladder neck

Figure 6.32 illustrates a common simple juxta-urethral fistula, with less than a half-circumferential defect.

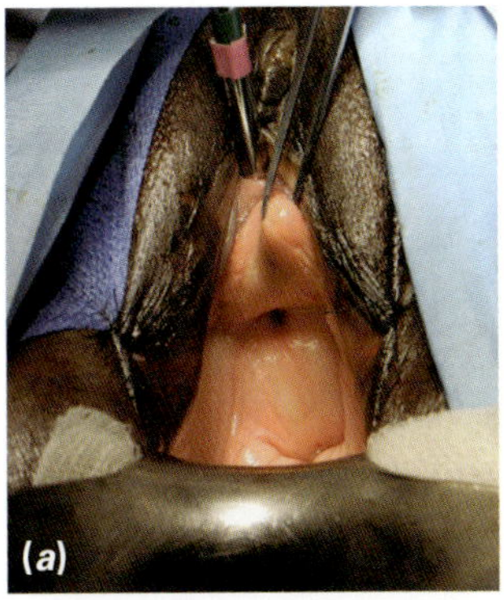

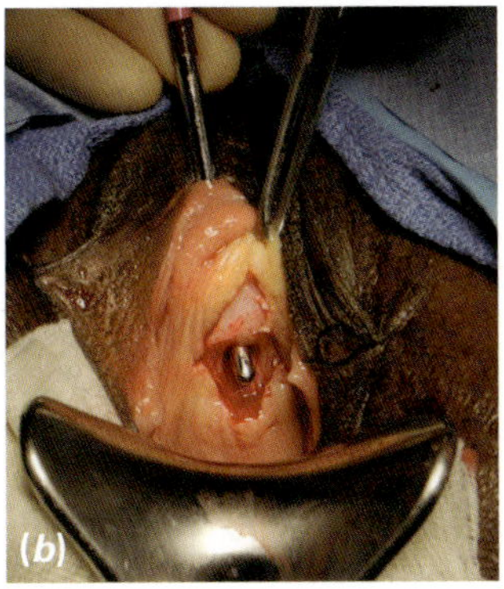

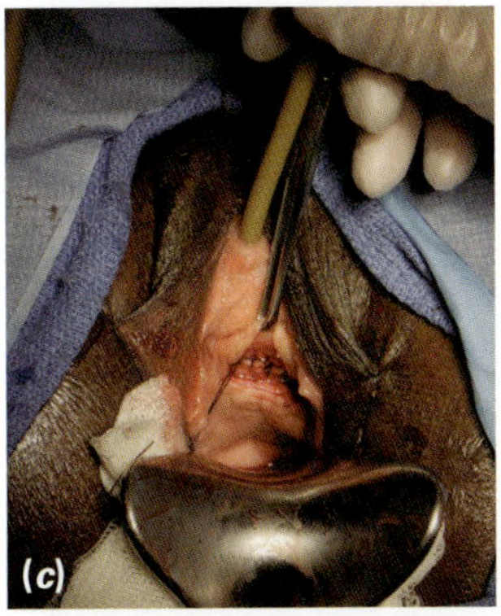

Figure 6.32 (*a*) As is often the case, the fistula is somewhat pulled up behind the symphysis. Head-down tilt of the operating table is essential for access. (*b*) The vaginal flaps have been reflected and the defect exposed. The distance from the external urethral orifice to the fistula is 3 cm. (*c*) The repair has been completed in one layer.

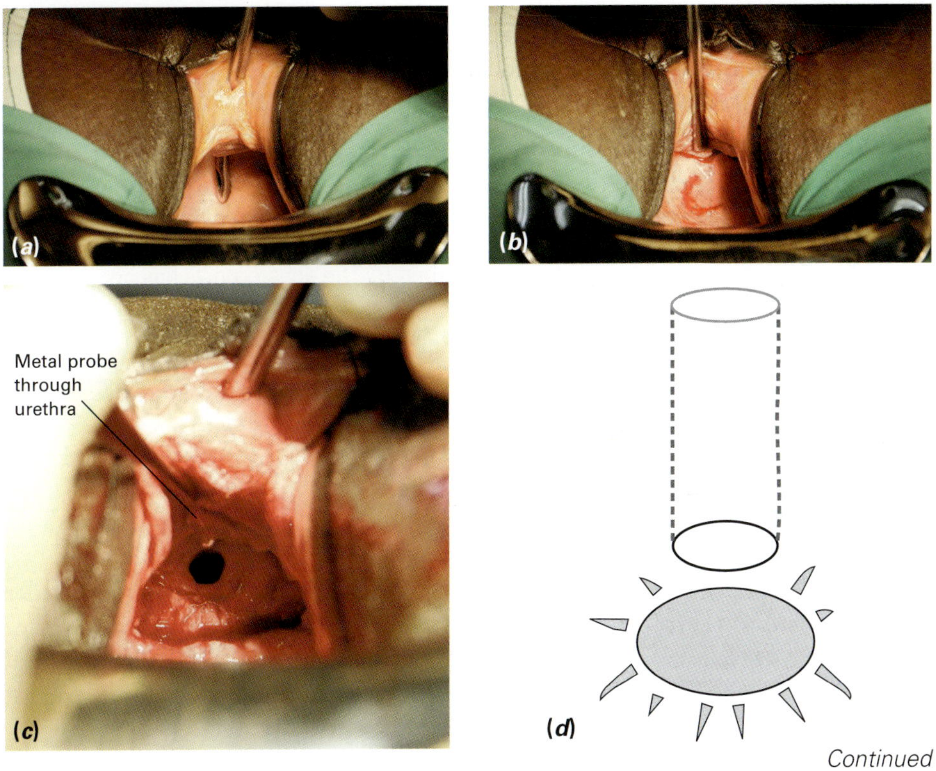

Continued

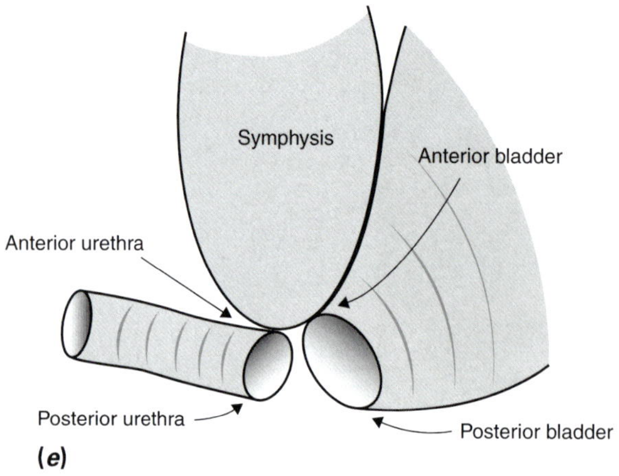

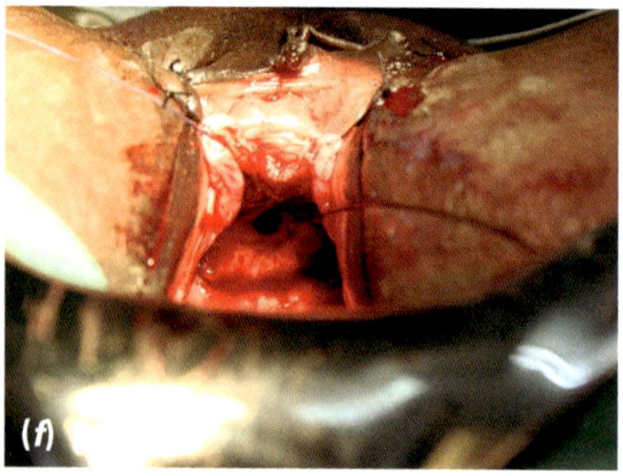

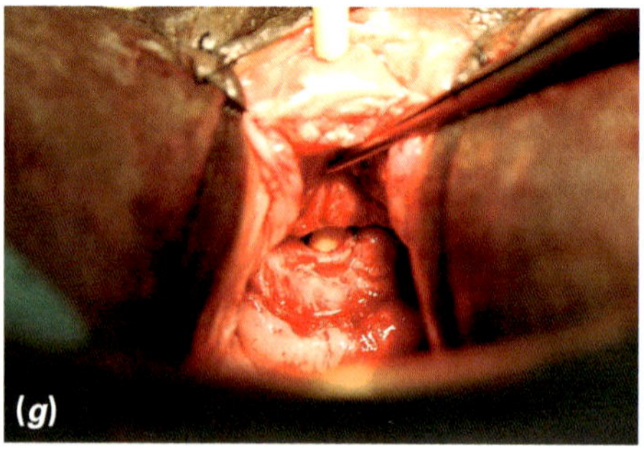

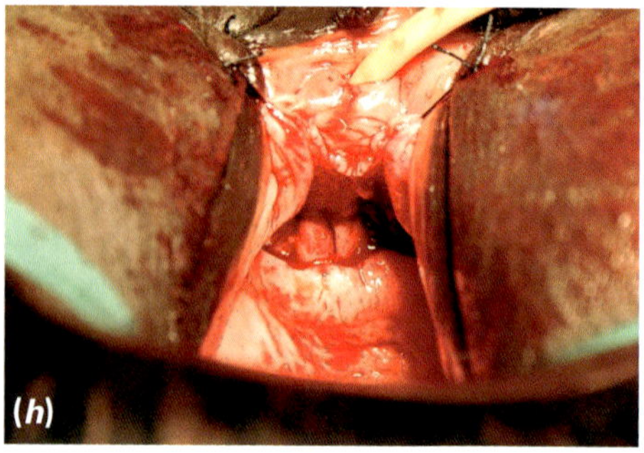

Figure 6.33 (*a*) The fistula is out of sight, being tethered behind the pubic bone. (*b*) After tilting the table, the defect is best exposed by placing the metal catheter through the fistula into the bladder. The first incision has been made. (*c*) The vaginal flaps have been separated. The hole seen is the entrance to the bladder. The metal catheter is in the urethra and can be just seen coming through the proximal end (arrowed). The bladder and urethra are just together on the deep aspect. (*d*) The surgeon's view of the defect. (*e*) A side view of the defect (for clarity, anterior and posterior are as indicated in this diagram). (*f*) A three-quarter anastomosis has been started by placing the two corner sutures at 2 and 10 o'clock. (*g*) Sutures have been placed at 3 and 9 o'clock, and the remaining posterior defect can be clearly seen over a catheter. (*h*) The anastomosis has been completed in one layer.

An almost-circumferential juxta-urethral fistula

A larger juxta-urethral fistula that is almost circumferential is shown in Figure 6.33.

Vertical closure

Another strategy for the non-circumferential bladder neck fistula is to consider vertical closure of the defect (Figure 6.34). This is possible only in about 10% of cases. The defect must be soft and mobile, and there must be no tension. Vertical closure will effectively increase urethral length, and may improve the prospect of continence.

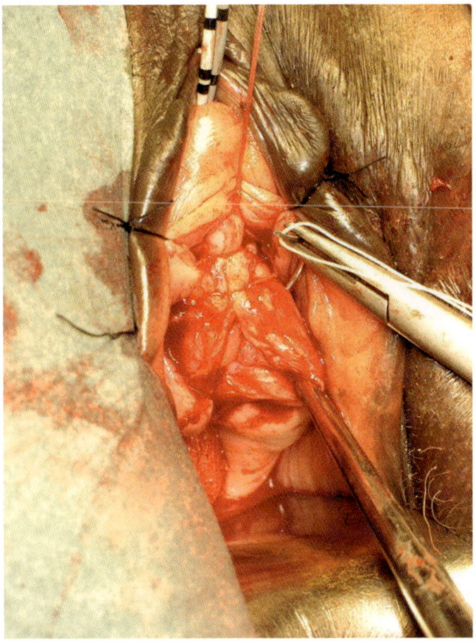

Figure 6.34 Vertical closure of a soft mobile juxta-urethral/mid-vaginal fistula.

Operative steps for circumferential fistulae

Where there is a clear separation of urethra and bladder, there are two options for repair:

- Incomplete mobilization and suture of the bladder to the pubic rami and urethra, leaving a gap on the anterior aspect.
- Complete mobilization of the bladder front, back and sides, followed by circumferential anastomosis to the urethra using a variety of methods to accommodate any discrepancy of size of the two ends. Where possible, an effort is made to reduce the diameter of the bladder where it is anastomosed to the urethra.

Incomplete mobilization

Incomplete mobilization (Figure 6.35) has, historically, been the method used to repair circumferential fistulae in the Addis Ababa Fistula Hospital, and is still practised by some surgeons trained there. The bladder is mobilized from the vagina and cervix only over its posterior and lateral aspects, until sufficient mobility has been obtained to bring the bladder directly to the antero-lateral boundaries of the bladder defect. This is, in effect, the undersurface of the pubic rami lateral to the urethra. Before this is done, a distal flap of vaginal epithelium will have been reflected off the pubic rami and urethra. Strong, small half-circle needles are needed to fix the bladder to the periosteum. The urethra is incorporated into this repair as the last step.

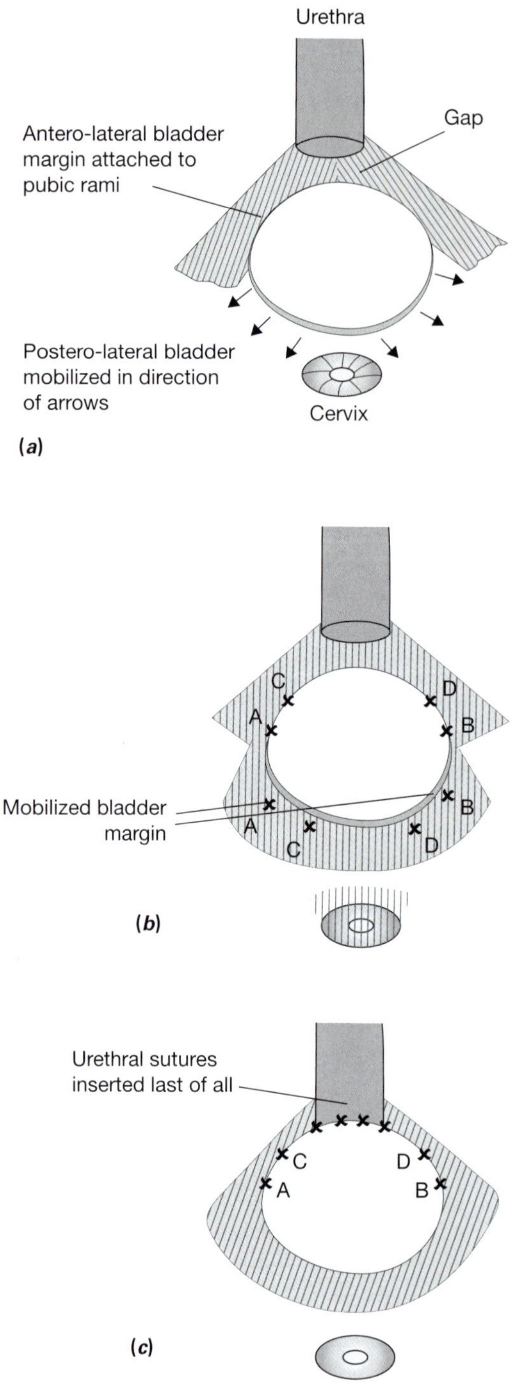

Figure 6.35 (*a*) Mobilization is only done postero-laterally (note that the ureters must be catheterized). (*b*) The mobilized bladder margin is sutured to the periostium/para-urethral area as indicated by the letters. (*c*) The urethral sutures are inserted last, using the centre of the posterior mobilized bladder.

Advantages of incomplete mobilization

- The operation may be easier to perform than a complete detachment and anastomosis. This will appeal to the novice surgeon or one working in difficult circumstances.
- A high rate of closure can be obtained.

Disadvantages of incomplete mobilization

- Stress incontinence may be unacceptably high.
- There is no muscle between the urethra and bladder on the anterior aspect and the urethra remains short.
- If the fistula breaks down in the corners (the most common place), the margin of the defect will be bone – an almost impossible situation to re-repair.
- Secondary operations for stress are often needed, and may be hazardous. The bladder immediately proximal to the urethra will have its anterior wall as a thin membrane of urothelium directly over the posterior symphysis. There is a risk of producing another fistula with a urethral and bladder base plication or with a rectus fascial sling operation. Opening the para-vesical space is a step used in many operations for stress.

Complete mobilization

The alternative of complete mobilization and circumferential anastomosis is recommended by most fistula experts, and is now increasingly used in the Addis Ababa Fistula Hospital.

After the usual posterior and lateral mobilization, the para-vesical space is freely entered. The bladder is dissected free of the pubic rami and symphysis. The retro-pubic space is entered, and the anterior bladder wall is freed so that it can be pulled down easily to reach the urethra. Sometimes, a suture may placed from the anterior wall to the back of the pubis to hold the bladder in place before beginning the anastomosis.

The anterior aspect of the urethra will be adherent under the symphysis. Scar in this region is excised, but no attempt is made to mobilize the urethra. The posterior and lateral aspects will already have been exposed by careful elevation of the distal vaginal flaps.

If the bladder opening is not too large and the urethra not short, the anastomosis can be completed end to end by bunching up the bladder side to make it fit. The anterior and two antero-lateral sutures are placed first, followed by two corner sutures – all of these take in a good bite of peri-urethral tissue. The posterior sutures are placed accurately through the urethral lumen. It is most important that bladder mucosa does not protrude through the suture line. Bites should be taken that invert the bladder mucosa.

Often, a mismatch between the diameter of the bladder opening and that of the urethra makes a straight end-to-end anastomosis impossible. The underlying principle in closure is to use the anterior and lateral bladder to wrap around the urethra and then to close the excess posterior bladder vertically. This has the effect of making the bladder lumen into a tube before joining the urethra. In the largest defects, this is not possible, because the postero-lateral margin containing the ureteric orifices cannot be mobilized enough to meet in the midline. The finished repair will then resemble an inverted 'V' or 'Y' (Figure 6.36). This also has the advantage of keeping the ureteric orifices in a more physiological position in relation to the new urethro-vesical junction.

Advantages of complete mobilization

- The urethro-vesical junction is now completely surrounded by muscle, and in many cases the bladder defect will have been converted to a tube, thus effectively lengthening the urethra. The incidence of postoperative stress incontinence may be reduced.
- A secondary stress operation can be more safely performed if required.

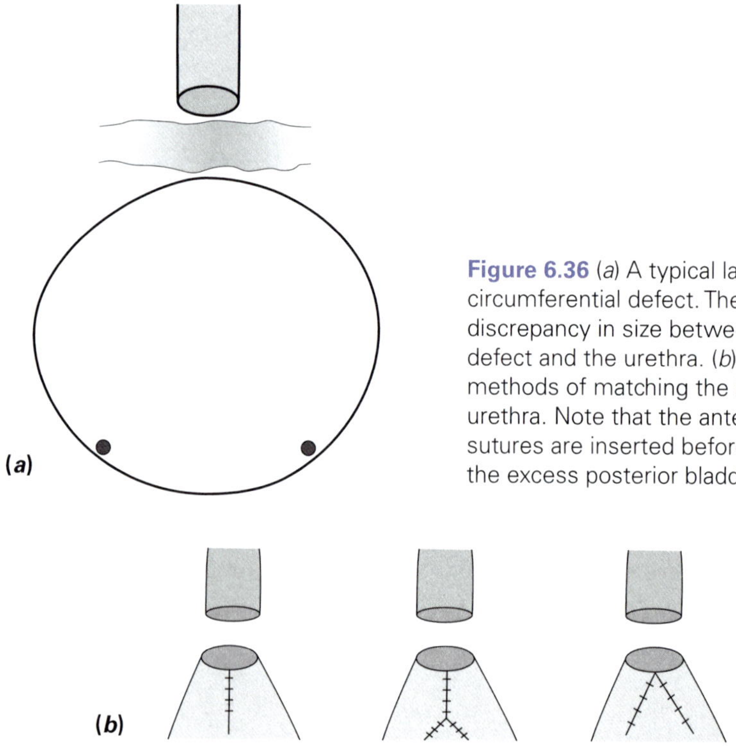

Figure 6.36 (*a*) A typical large circumferential defect. There is a large discrepancy in size between the bladder defect and the urethra. (*b*) The three methods of matching the bladder to the urethra. Note that the anterior and lateral sutures are inserted before dealing with the excess posterior bladder.

Disadvantages of complete mobilization

- The anastomosis is technically more demanding, and if not well done may be more prone to break down.

A complete mobilization illustrated

In the case shown in Figure 6.37, there is a small gap between the urethra and bladder (more evident on palpation than inspection). The bladder will be detached from the back of the pubis. There is only a slight discrepancy in size between urethra and bladder lumina.

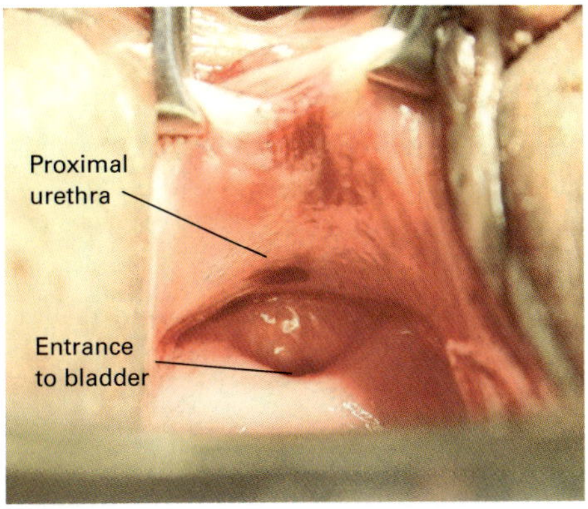

Figure 6.37 (*a*) The proximal urethra is seen detached from the bladder.

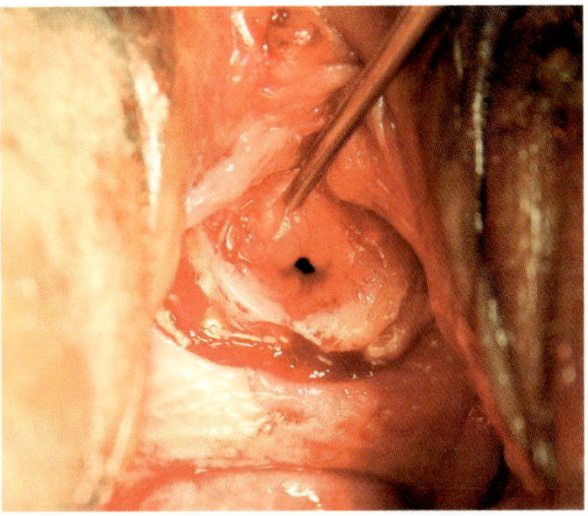

Figure 6.37 (*b*) The bladder has been mobilized all round and the anterior bladder is pulled down to demonstrate its mobility.

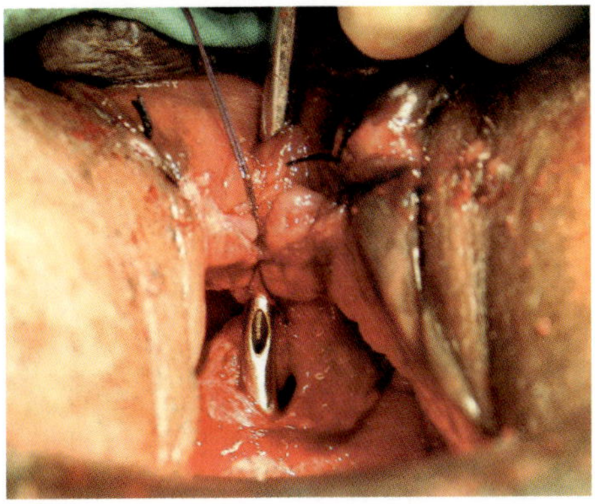

Figure 6.37 (*c*) The anterior (12 o'clock) midline suture has been inserted. The knot will be inside the lumen. Note the metal catheter through the urethra.

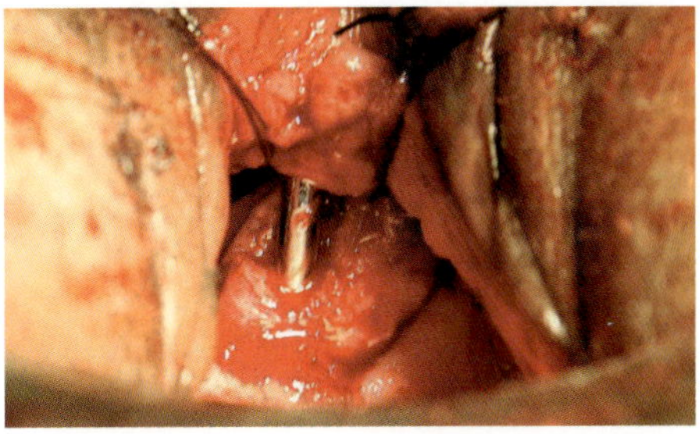

Figure 6.37 (*d*) Two antero-lateral sutures (2 and 10 o'clock) have now been inserted.

Continued

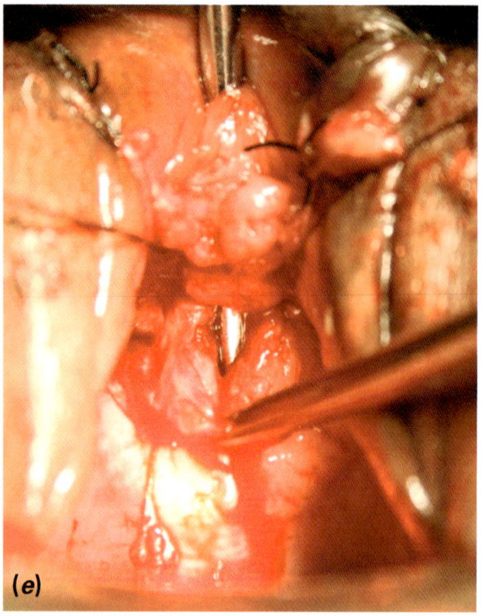

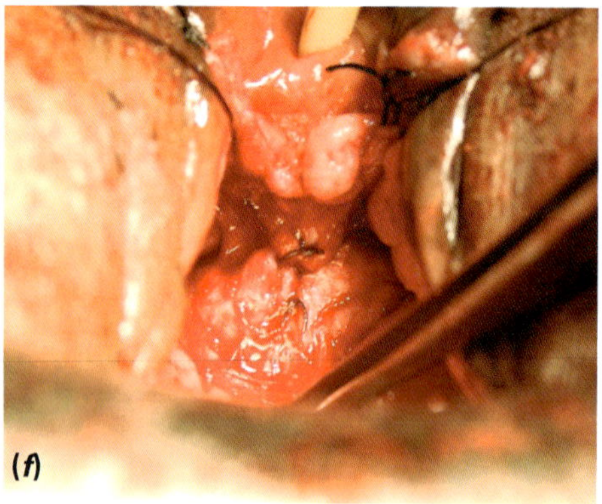

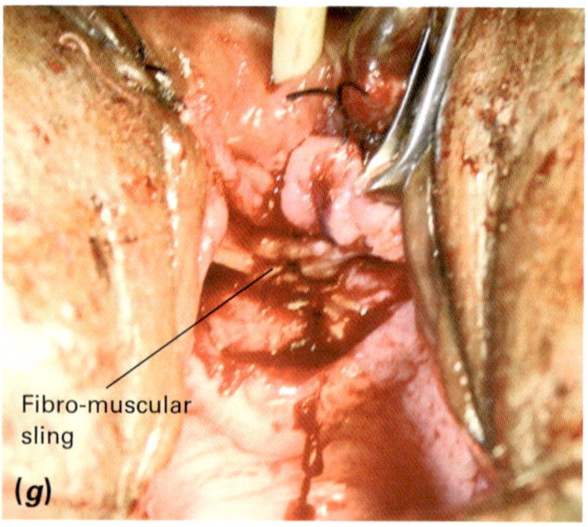

Figure 6.37 (*e*) The posterior half of the anastomosis remains to be sutured. (*f*) The anastomosis is completed using a small vertical extension because of the discrepancy in size. (*g*) Because the urethra was less than 2.5 cm in diameter, a fibro-muscular sling has been made.

Circumferential anastomosis

Figure 6.38 shows an example of circumferential anastomosis in a large fistula.

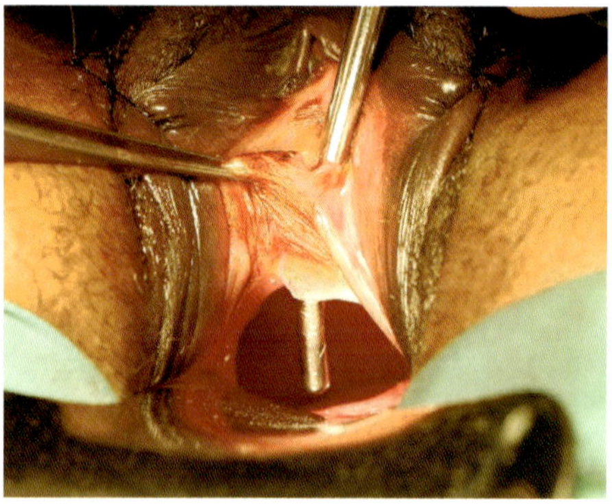

Figure 6.38 (*a*) A large circumferential fistula with a 2.5 cm urethra.

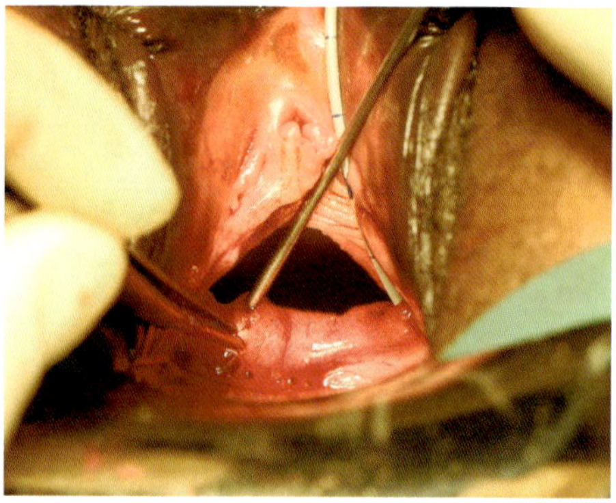

Figure 6.38 (*b*) The left ureteric orifice has been catheterized and the right has been identified with a probe.

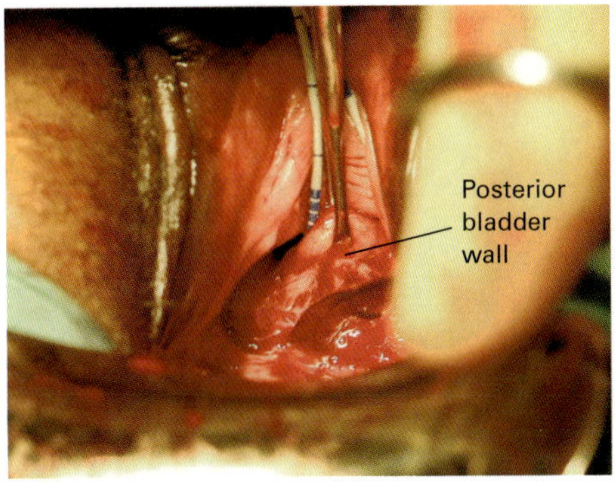

Figure 6.38 (*c*) The posterior bladder margin is held up as it is mobilized off the vagina and cervix.

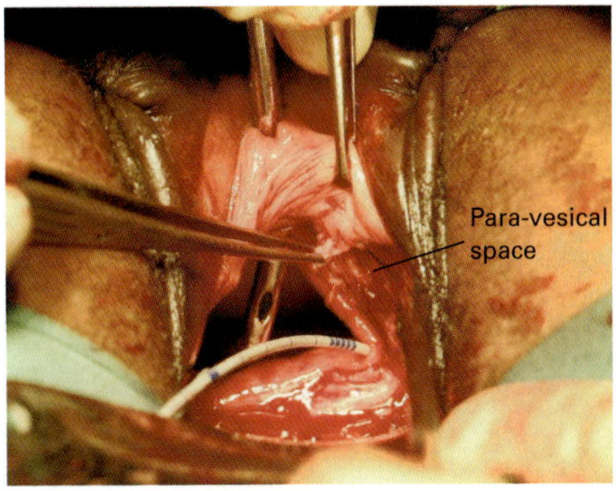

Figure 6.38 (*d*) The para-vesical space is entered on the left. Then the distal vaginal flap is elevated.

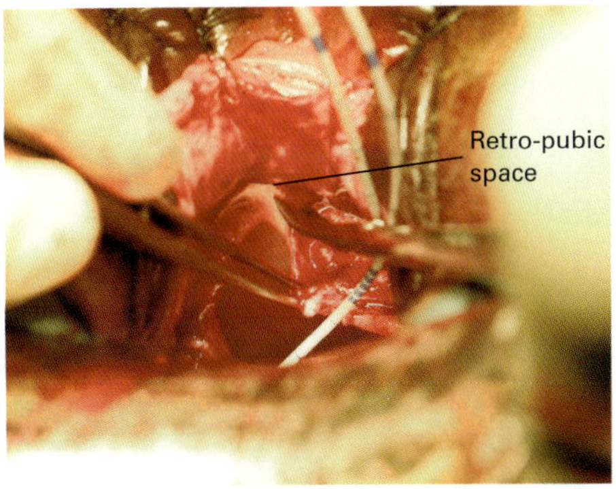

Figure 6.38 (*e*) The left antero-lateral bladder is dissected from the pubic rami.

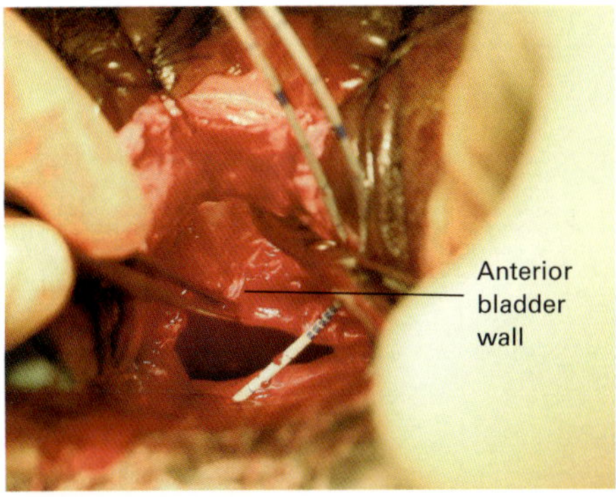

Figure 6.38 (*f*) The scissors are entering the retro-pubic space to free up the anterior bladder wall.

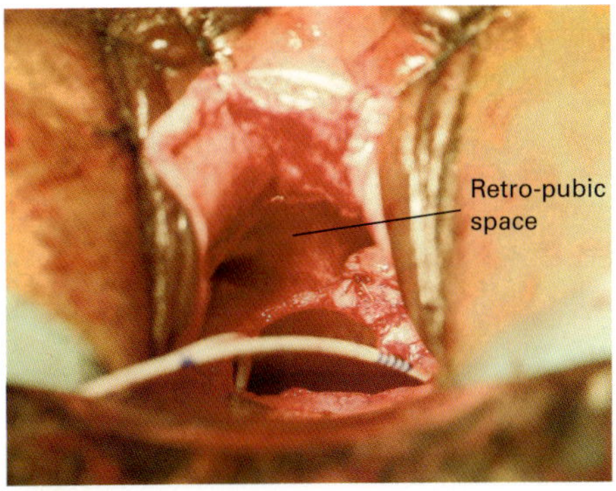

Figure 6.38 (*g*) The retro-pubic space is open and the anterior bladder wall is mobile.

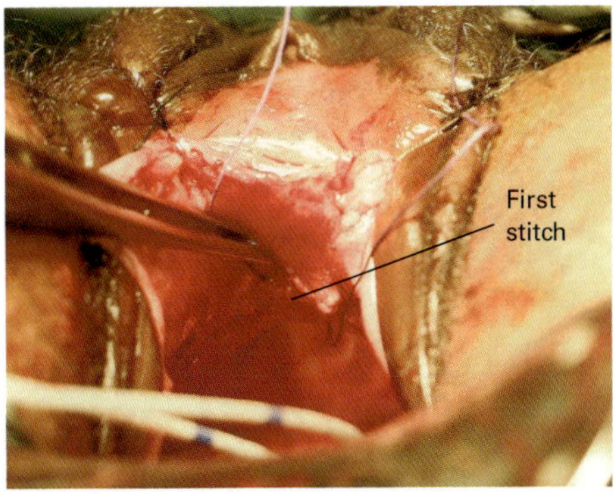

Figure 6.38 (*h*) The first suture has been placed into the periosteum adjacent to the anterior aspect of the urethra.

Continued

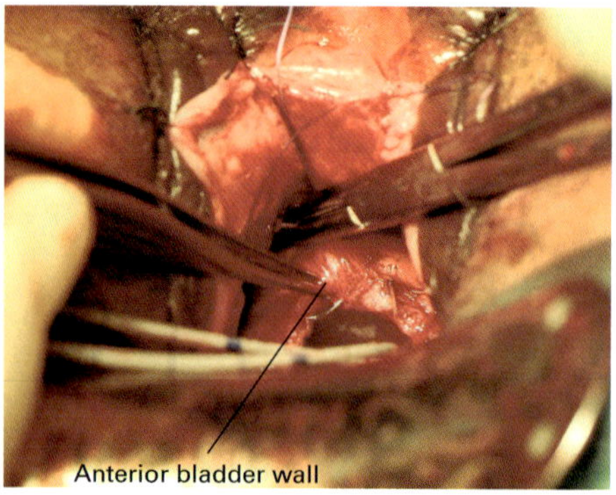

Figure 6.38 (*i*) Now a good bite is taken of the anterior bladder wall in the midline.

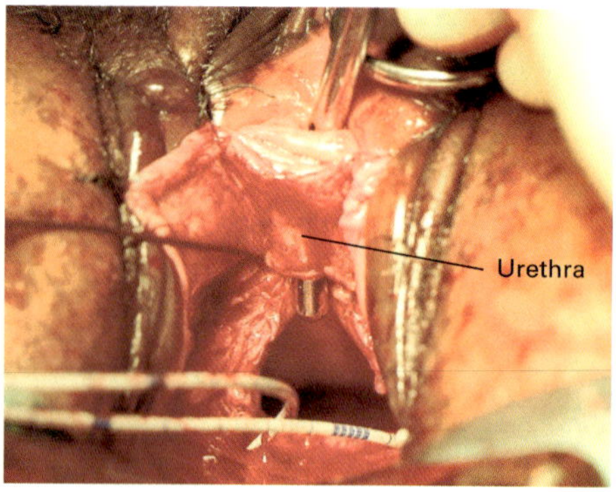

Figure 6.38 (*j*) The suture has been tied to approximate the bladder and urethra anteriorly (12 o'clock stitch).

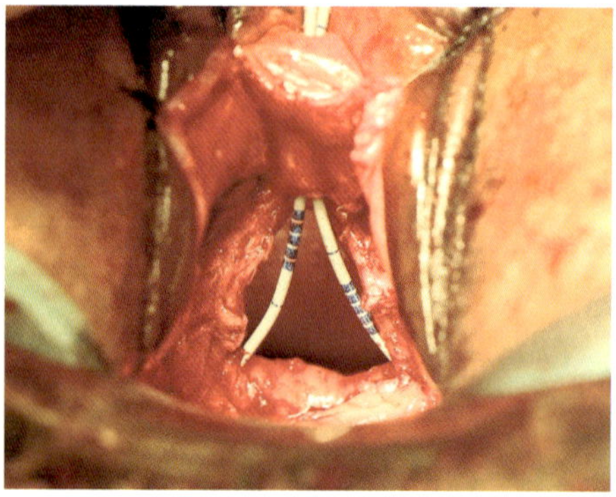

Figure 6.38 (*k*) Both ureteric catheters are pulled through the urethra.

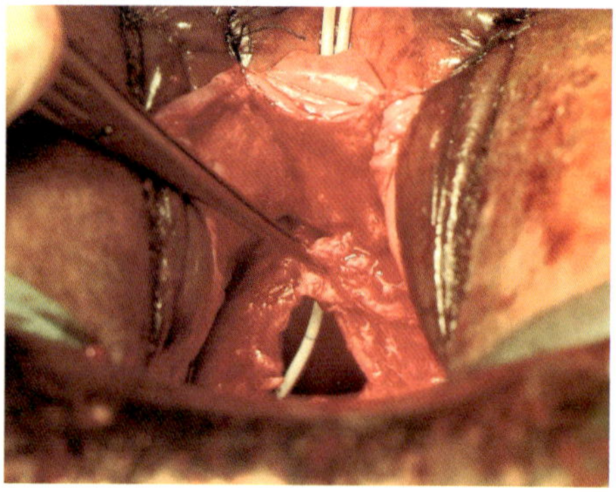

Figure 6.38 (*l*) The antero-lateral bladder wall is used to complete a circumferential anastomosis.

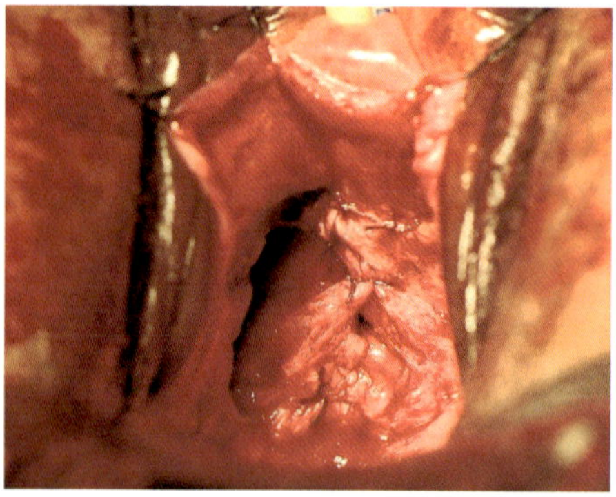

Figure 6.38 (*m*) The remaining bladder is closed vertically.

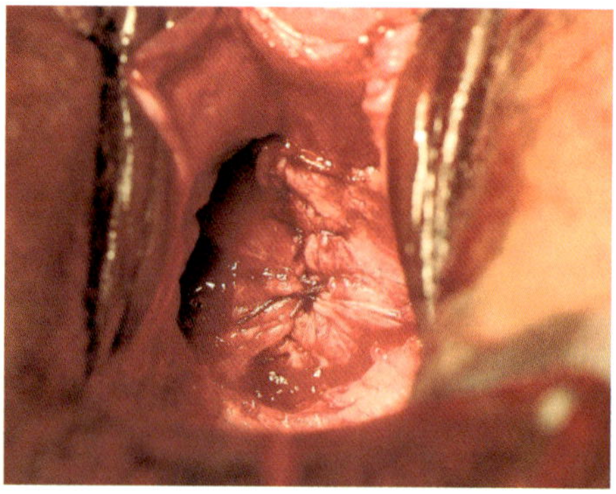

Figure 6.38 (*n*) The anastomosis is now complete.

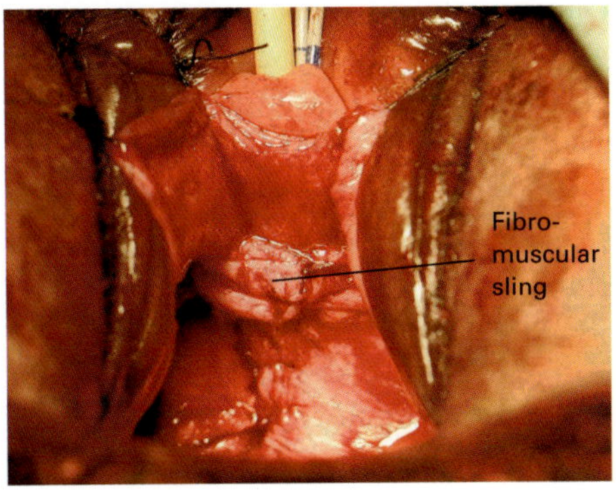

Figure 6.38 (*o*) A fibro-muscular sling of pubo-coccygeus is added to support the urethra.

Incomplete versus complete mobilization

Unfortunately, there are no hard data to allow a comparison of closure and incontinence rates between the two methods, but the consensus of opinion among the most experienced fistula surgeons is that a complete detachment and anastomosis does give better results. It makes sense to restore muscular continuity between bladder and urethra front and back.

It must be appreciated that, although the anastomosis can be easily performed in some cases as shown in our illustrations, in many others (which are almost impossible to photograph) the operation is quite demanding and requires a high degree of skill and judgement. It is probably only full-time fistula surgeons who have the experience to achieve good results with this group, as illustrated in a published series by Andrew Browning.[1] In a consecutive series of 321 new patients, 24% were classified as having circumferential fistulae. Of these 77 cases, 5 were inoperable as there was no bladder to repair. Of the 72 operated upon, the breakdown rate was 2.7%, but stress incontinence was high at 47%. In many, it was mild, and others were dry with a urethral plug. Almost all the circumferential fistulae were treated by complete detachment and re-anastomosis.

I have not been able to match these results for closure in my own series, although I only classify 10% of my patients as circumferential. For these, I always used to do an incomplete detachment as I had learnt at the Addis Ababa Fistula Hospital, but over the last few years I have increasingly performed a complete detachment with circumferential anastomosis. My series is quite small and I have not yet been able to demonstrate any significant improvement in my results, but I still believe that complete detachment is the right procedure whenever possible.

For those with less experience, we believe that there is still a place for incomplete detachment, provided that the gap is not too large and there is no expert available to take on the case.

Ureteric involvement

The larger the fistula and the closer it is to the cervix, the greater is the chance of ureteric involvement (Figure 6.39). During every fistula repair, one must keep in mind the position of the ureteric orifices. For small fistulae at the bladder neck, the orifices should not be close, but it must be borne in mind that what was once a large defect involving most of the anterior vaginal wall and bladder base will have contracted in the first 3 months (Figure 6.40). Thus, the anterior wall will be short and the ureteric orifices may be close to the fistula edge, even though the defect

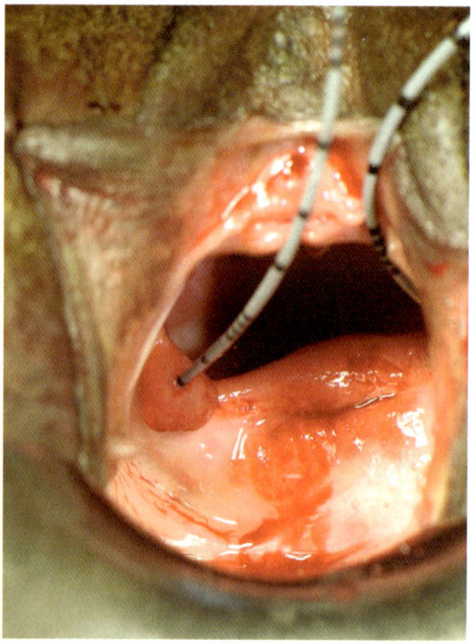

Figure 6.39 Ureter on the edge of a large fistula.

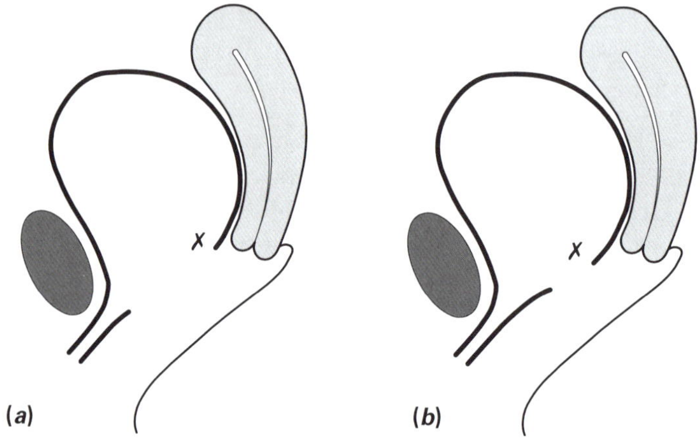

Figure 6.40 (*a*) Initial size of defect. (*b*) Size 3 months later. The cross marks the position of the ureter.

appears to start at the urethro-vesical junction. Likewise, a small defect in the region of the cervix may have been much larger at first, and subsequent contraction will have brought the ureters close to the edge of the defect.

There may be complex ureteric involvement in large circumferential fistulae. The distal end of the ureter may be involved in the ischaemic process and the uretero-vesical junction may slough away as a result, leaving the ureter draining directly into the vagina rather than into the bladder. In this case, there are three options for repair:

- If the ureter is just on or outside the edge of the bladder mucosa then, after catheterization of the ureter and sufficient mobilization of the tissues, it is possible to merely fold the ureter (containing a ureteric catheter) into the bladder as part of the repair. The ureteric catheter needs to remain in place to splint open the healing tissues for about 7 days.
- Occasionally the ureter is too far from the edge to be merely 'folded' in. In this case, it can be catheterized and then mobilized a little off the pelvic side wall. It can then be brought into the bladder at a higher level than the repair through a separate stab incision. The ureter is secured in place by 3/0 sutures through its muscularis and the bladder wall. The ureteric catheter should stay in for 12–14 days.
- Exceptionally, the ureter is too far from the bladder to be re-implanted. The options are to implant the ureter into the bladder by an abdominal approach at the same operation, or to catheterize it for 2 weeks and defer the re-implantation.

It must be appreciated that, if the last two steps are required, there is usually such severe damage that the outcomes are poor.

Other strategies for dealing with the ureters will be described in the section on juxta- and intra-cervical fistulae later in this chapter.

As stress incontinence is such a problem after repair of juxta-urethral and circumferential fistulae, some measures that can be taken to reduce its incidence are described in the next section.

OPERATIVE STEPS TO REDUCE THE INCIDENCE OF STRESS INCONTINENCE

We know the factors that predispose to incontinence from a multivariant analysis of patients in Ethiopia by Andrew Browning.[2] These are:

- involvement of the urethra (types 2–4 in Goh's classification) – the shorter the urethra, the greater the stress
- large fistulae
- vaginal scarring sufficient to prevent insertion of a speculum without vaginotomy

- small bladder volume post repair (<150 cm^3).

Most important is loss of length and quality of urethral tissue, so any measures that can be taken to improve this should be taken. These fall into three groups:

- lengthening procedures
- repair of the pubo-cervical fascia where possible
- urethral support with a fibro-muscular sling.

Lengthening procedures

In a series of patients with severe post-repair stress incontinence from Andrew Browning, the average urethral length was 1.4 cm, which is less than half the normal length of 3–4 cm. Thus, anything that can be done to lengthen the urethra should help.

As mentioned in the section above on juxta-urethral and circumferential fistulae, it is possible in some cases to fashion the bladder side of the anastomosis into a tube with a diameter approaching that of the urethra. This is done by joining the anterior wall and sides of the bladder to the urethral remnant and closing the remaining defect in a vertical direction.

As also mentioned in the previous section, vertical closure of the defect is possible in a few cases.

Repair of the pubo-cervical fascia

The pubo-cervical fascia is a sheet that originates from the arcus tendinus on the pelvic side wall. It is a fascial sling that supports the urethra, the urethro-vesical junction and bladder base. It is disrupted by the ischaemic process, and attempts to repair this damage are worthwhile, even though it may appear insubstantial. Some surgeons make a quite extensive dissection over the bladder base to identify the fascia and pull it together in the midline, thus supporting and elevating the new urethro-vesical junction (Figure 6.41). This is really just a radical plication of the distal bladder.

Urethral support with a fibro-muscular sling (pubo-coccygeal sling)

A review by Andrew Browning of 318 consecutive patients successfully repaired at the Addis Ababa Fistula Hospital in the year 2000 showed an immediate postoperative incontinence rate of 33%. Repair was by simple closure, with a fat graft added in most cases. This was a much higher figure for incontinence than had previously been recognized, and he started to use a fibro-muscular sling in high-risk cases, i.e. those with a shortened urethra (<2.5 cm from the external urethral orifice,

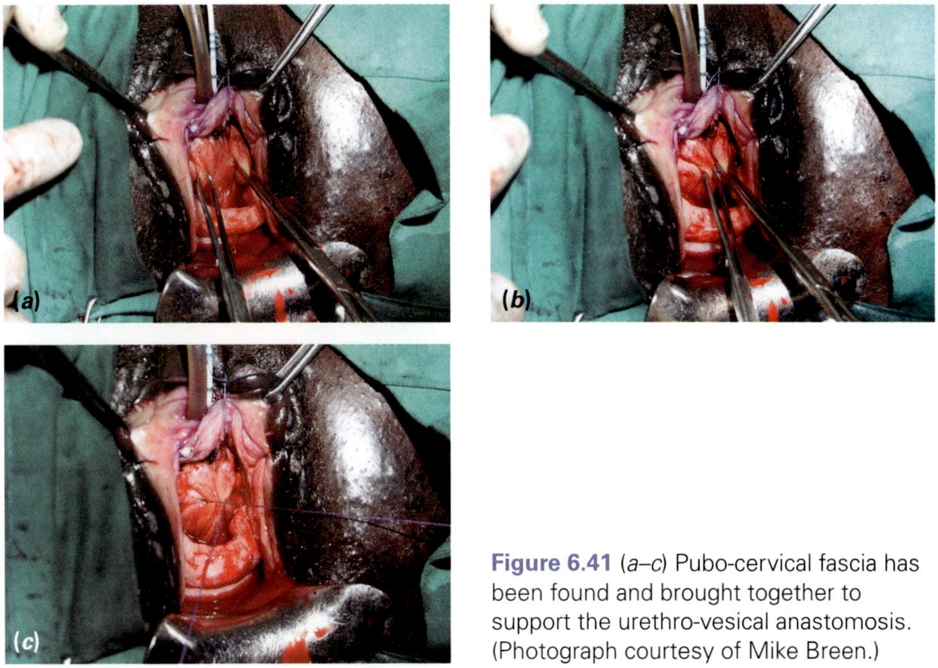

Figure 6.41 (*a–c*) Pubo-cervical fascia has been found and brought together to support the urethro-vesical anastomosis. (Photograph courtesy of Mike Breen.)

Goh's type 3 and 4). Since this was adopted in his routine practice, the rate of postoperative stress incontinence has been reduced to 18%.[3]

The exact nature of the tissues used to make the sling is open to debate, but is generally considered to be pubo-coccygeal muscle.

The procedure is best understood by referring to the diagram and photographs shown in Figure 6.42. The lateral ends of the vaginal incision that was made around the fistula are extended a little downwards in the axis of the vagina. The vaginal skin is elevated so as to expose some fibro-muscular tissue under the pubic rami. The belly of fibro-muscular tissue that can be felt in this area is grasped with Allis forceps. A cut is made below with scissors so as to elevate a broad rectangular block of tissue attached anteriorly under the pubic arch. The same procedure is performed on the other side, and then the two sides are sutured together in the midline beneath the urethra with two interrupted sutures. If the dissection has been taken high enough, the sling should wrap around the urethra in a gentle 'U' shape.

Unfortunately, in many of the worst cases, the pubo-coccygeal muscle has been destroyed and replaced by fibrosis. The sling will then be mostly scar, but may still give some support.

We use this sling in most patients with fistulae that are less than 2.5 cm from the external urethral orifice. We may also be influenced by the quality of the urethra, using the sling when the urethra is thin and also sometimes adding it to longer urethras when an obvious urethral leak is noticed on dye testing.

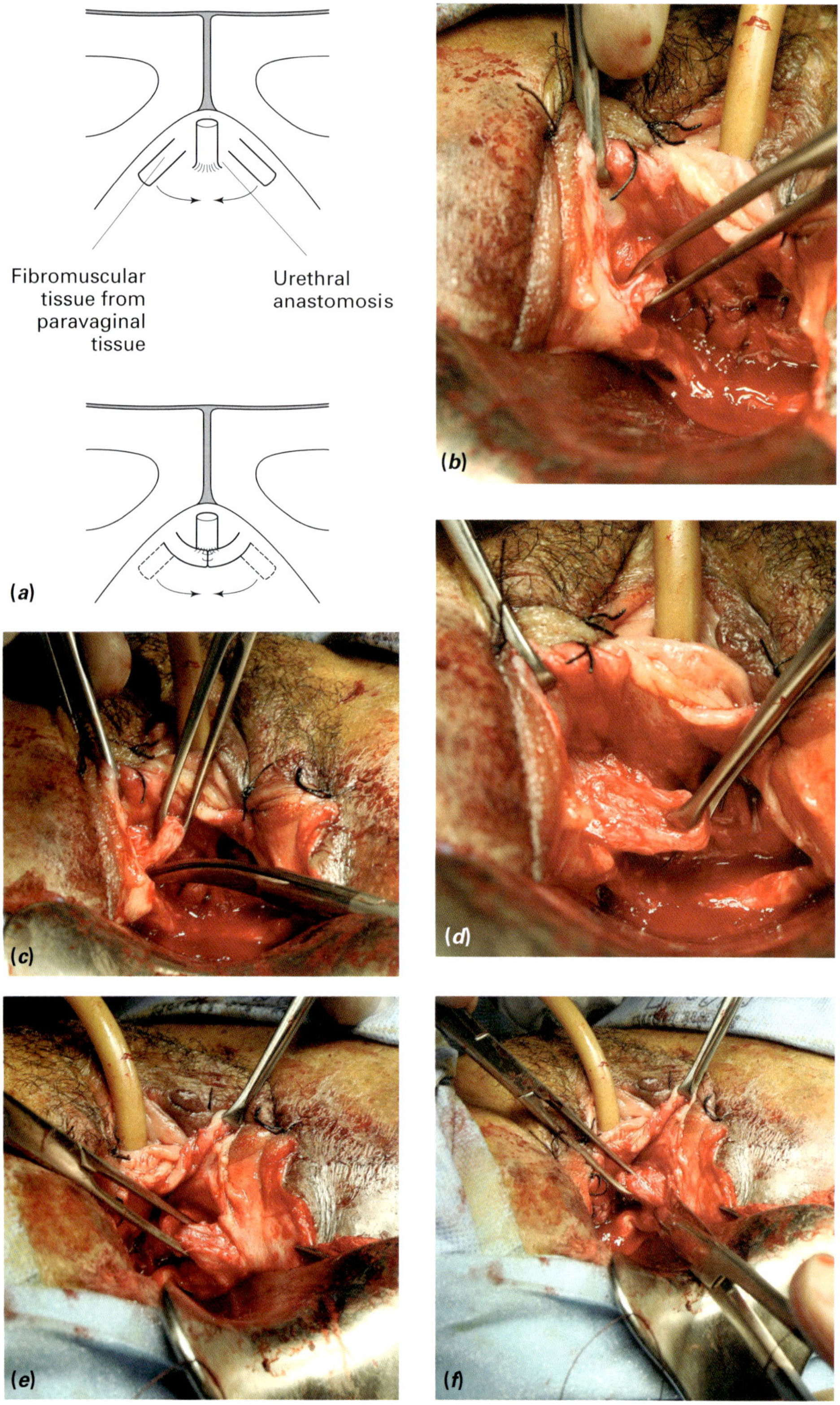
Fibromuscular tissue from paravaginal tissue
Urethral anastomosis
(a)
(b)
(c)
(d)
(e)
(f)

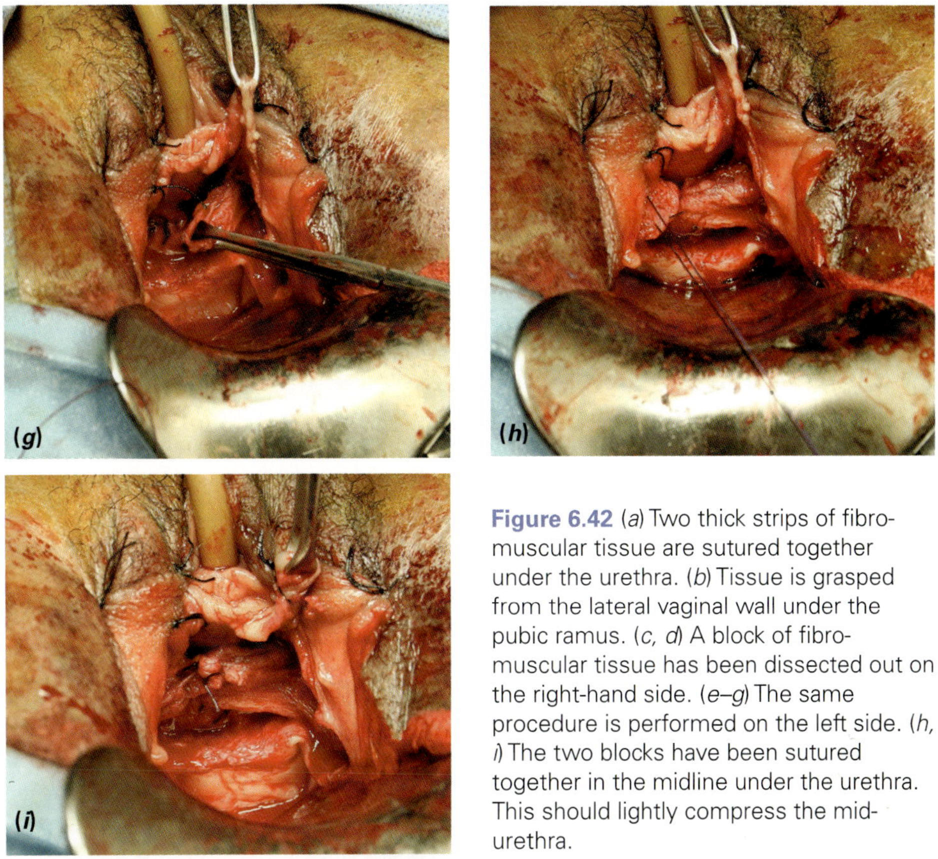

Figure 6.42 (*a*) Two thick strips of fibromuscular tissue are sutured together under the urethra. (*b*) Tissue is grasped from the lateral vaginal wall under the pubic ramus. (*c, d*) A block of fibromuscular tissue has been dissected out on the right-hand side. (*e–g*) The same procedure is performed on the left side. (*h, i*) The two blocks have been sutured together in the midline under the urethra. This should lightly compress the mid-urethra.

JUXTA- AND INTRA-CERVICAL FISTULAE

A fistula in the region of the cervix is often called a juxta-cervical fistula. Fistulae in this region can be divided into three main types:

1. The fistula is just distal to the cervix, and both distal and proximal margins are visible.
2. The distal margin can be visualized, but the proximal margin is out of sight in the cervical canal (the anterior lip of which is often split open)
3. The fistula cannot be seen at all, i.e. it is entirely intra-cervical.

Beginners should attempt only small juxta-cervical fistulae that can be easily exposed. The proximal margin between the fistula and the cervix must be clearly seen. Those that extend into the cervical canal can be challenging to close.

The general principle in repairing fistulae close to the cervix is to begin the flap splitting on the distal margin. This is exposed by upward traction with two Allis forceps applied close to the distal fistula margin. The bladder wall is supported by a metal catheter through the urethra and fistula. A small vertical incision is made through the vagina down to the fistula margin and then taken round the distal margins to the sides, where a small lateral extension may be made. The antero-lateral flaps are developed, keeping just under the vaginal mucosa. It is easy to stray into the bladder wall. These flaps are then sutured up to the labia. The postero-lateral dissection towards the cervix must be carried out with extreme caution, staying just under the vagina. The ureter is very much at risk where it runs in the wall of the bladder. It should, if possible, already have been catheterized.

An easy case

A type 1 case is shown in Figure 6.43. As a general rule if the fistula is very small (<0.5 cm) and in the midline then the ureters should not be at risk. However, if one can see into the bladder then they should always be identified. Babcock forceps should be used to evert the bladder – toothed forceps cause bleeding. Intravenous furosemide 20 mg should be administered if there is still difficulty.

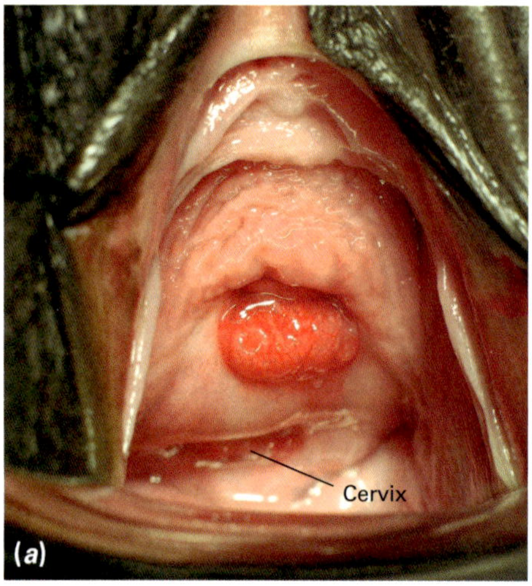

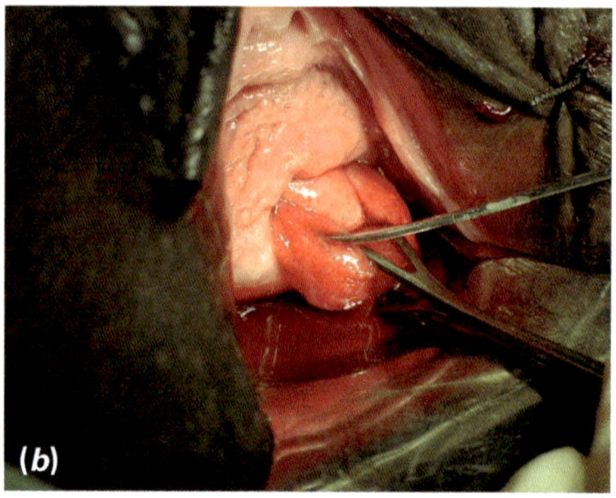

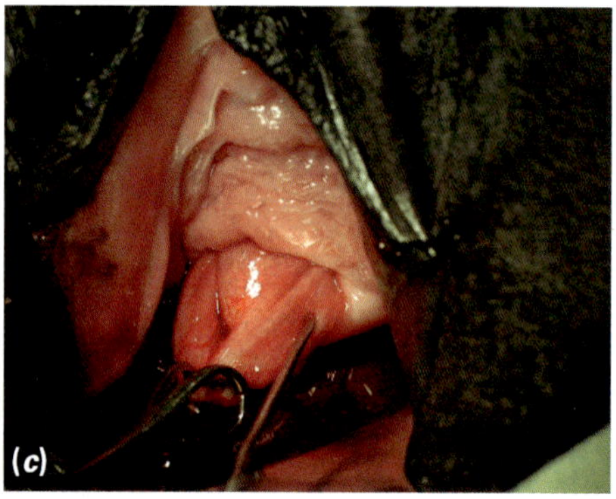

Figure 6.43 (*a*) There is a clear space between this fistula and the cervix. The distance from the external urethral orifice to the distal fistula margin is 5 cm. (*b*) Babcock forceps are used to evert the bladder. (*c*) Both ureteric orifices have been found closer to the margin than might have been expected.

Intermediate examples

Figures 6.44 and 6.45 show two intermediate examples.

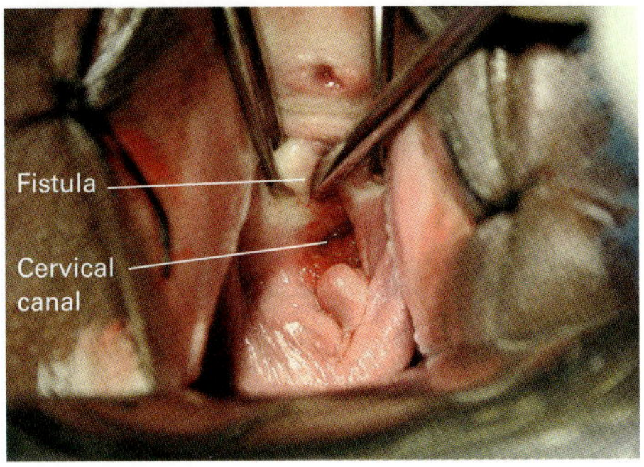

Figure 6.44 This fistula demonstrated by the metal catheter is separated from the cervical canal by a thin septum. Most of the anterior cervix has been lost.

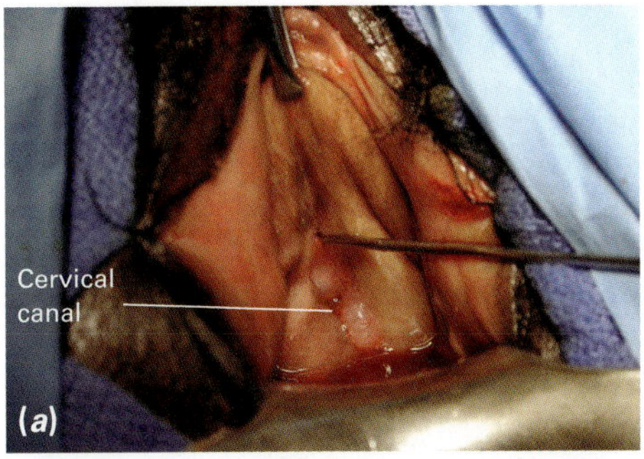

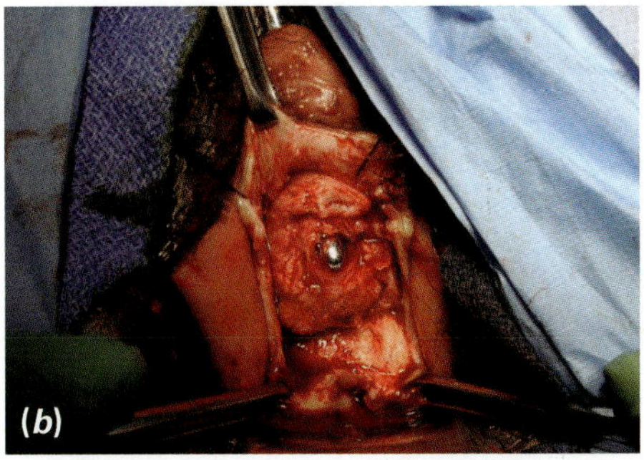

Figure 6.45 (*a*) This juxta-cervical fistula is very close to the cervical canal. (*b*) In the same case, the vagina has been reflected and the bladder dissected off the cervix to expose the small defect. It would be impossible to expose the ureters unless the defect were to be enlarged, but there is no need to do this, as the patient will not be at risk with such a small defect. It can be closed with three sutures.

Combined juxta-/intra-cervical fistulae

An example of a combined juxta-/intra-cervical fistula is shown in Figure 6.46. If the ureters are not easily found in this sort of case, a Langenbeck or Sims speculum should be used to expose the interior of the bladder (Figure 6.47).

Figure 6.48 shows a juxta-cervical fistula that extends high up into an open cervical canal. If the cervix does not come down well, cases like this can be very challenging to close and impossible to photograph. They should be left for experienced surgeons.

The incidence of this combined juxta-/intra-cervical fistula may vary from place to place. In one hospital in Uganda, 75% of fistula patients have been delivered by caesarean section, so this injury is seen quite often. Conversely, in Ethiopia, where only 15% have had a caesarean section, it is uncommon.

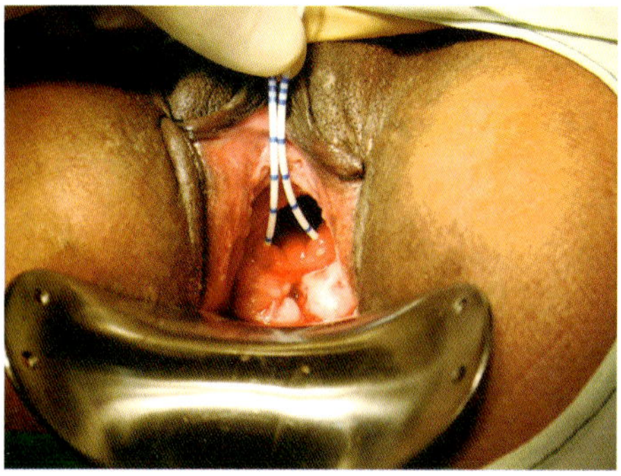

Figure 6.46 (*a*) The split anterior cervix can be seen. Both ureters are catheterized.

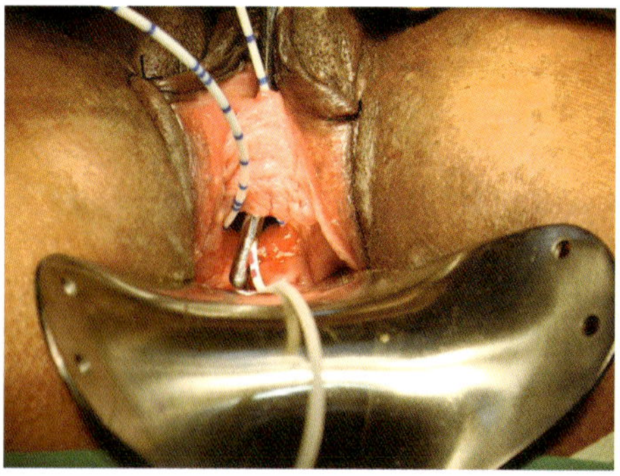

Figure 6.46 (*b*) The ureteric catheters are withdrawn through the urethra by passing the catheter into the eye of a metal catheter. This is an atraumatic method.

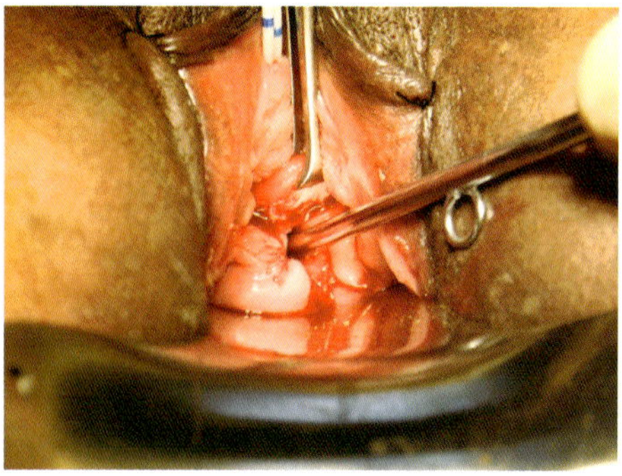

Figure 6.46 (*c*) To help the dissection between bladder and cervix, a metal catheter has been inserted into the cervical canal. The proximal bladder margin is held in the Allis forceps.

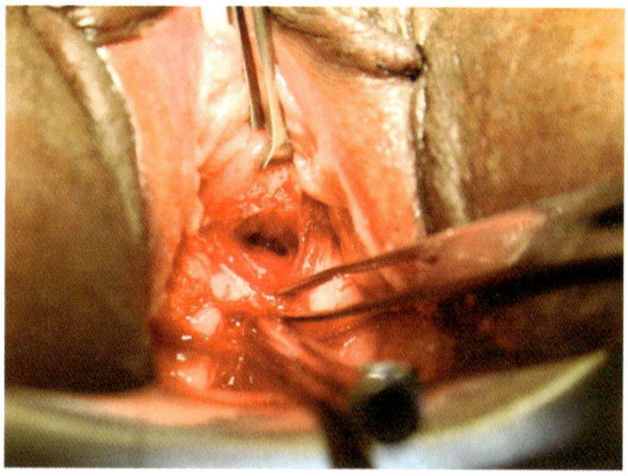

Figure 6.46 (*d*) The avascular plane between the cervix and bladder is opened (note the metal catheter in the cervical canal).

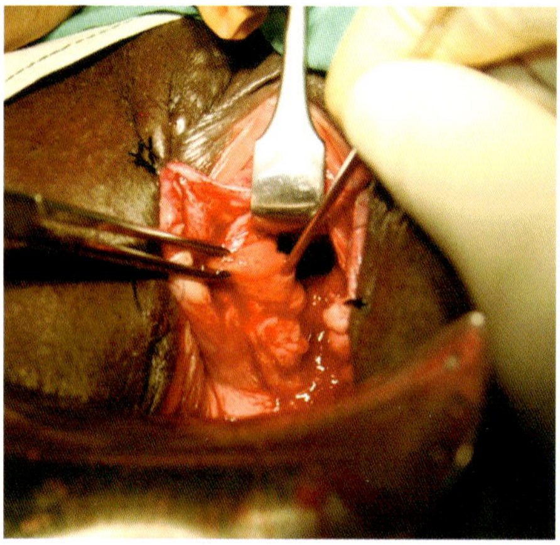

Figure 6.47 A Langenbeck retractor placed inside the fistula often aids in identification of the ureters.

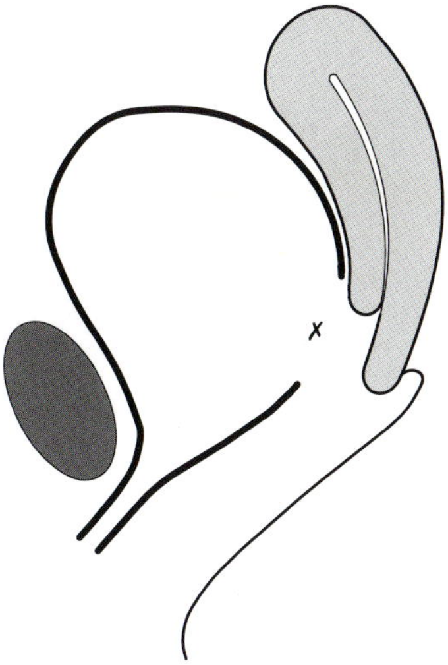

Figure 6.48 (*a*) A combined juxta-/intra-cervical fistula. The anterior cervical canal is missing. The approximate position of the ureteric orifice is indicated by the cross.

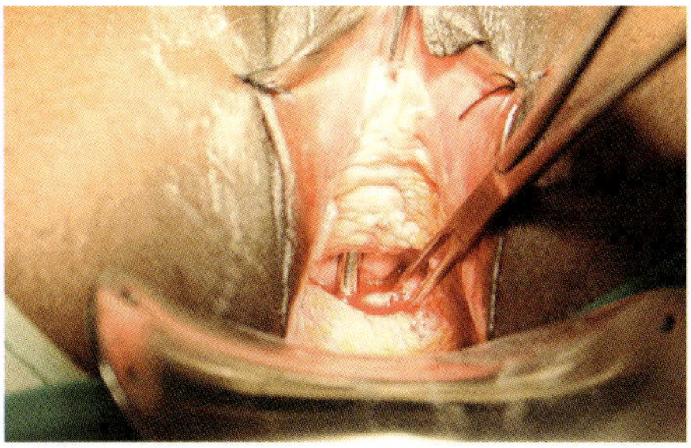

Figure 6.48 (*b*) Initial view. The proximal margin is far out of sight.

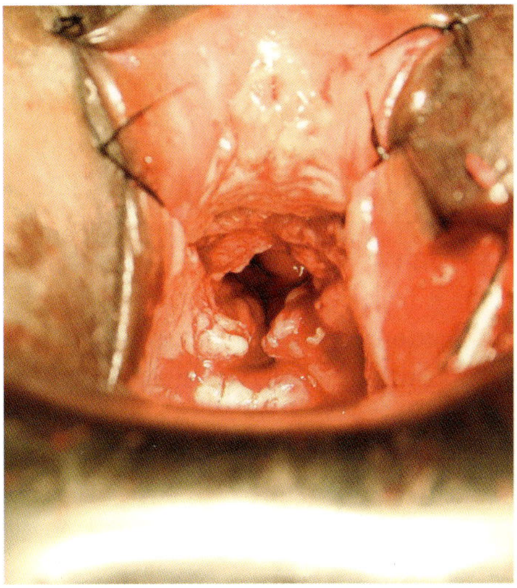

Figure 6.48 (*c*) The distal dissection has been completed and antero-lateral flaps sutured out of the way.

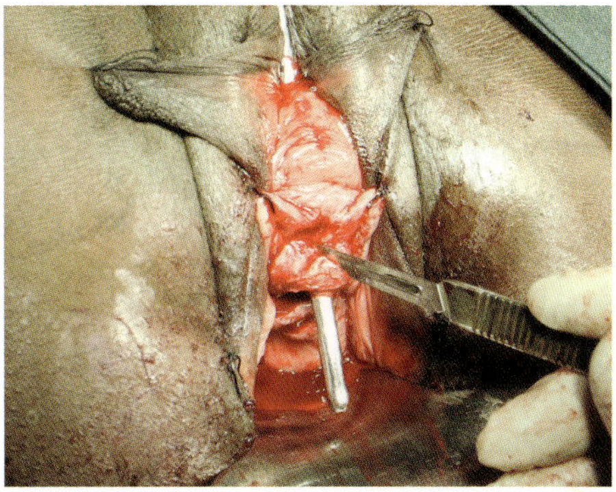

Figure 6.48 (*d*) The ureters are often distal to the fistula. If they cannot be found by everting the fistula margin then a cut should be made distally as shown to enlarge the fistula. The bladder defect is almost always closed vertically.

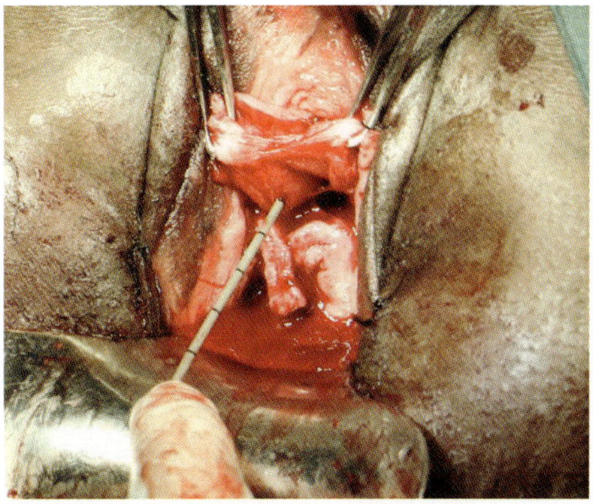

Figure 6.48 (*e*) The cut margins are everted to expose the ureteric orifices. It will also now be possible to insert a Sims speculum to see the proximal limit of the defect.

Continued

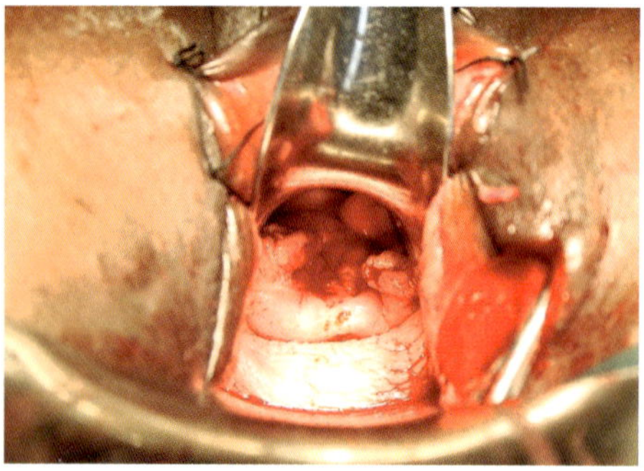

Figure 6.48 (*f*) A Sims speculum is placed inside the fistula to show the defect extending up the cervical canal. The latter is wide open. With the speculum in place and the ureters identified, the bladder must be dissected from the cervix up to the apex of the defect.

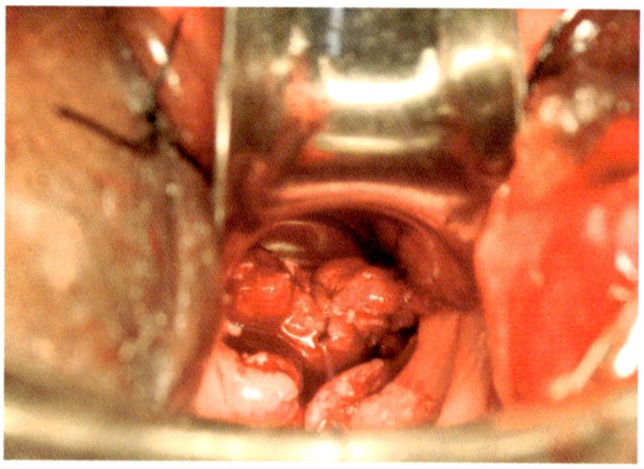

Figure 6.48 (*g*) The bladder margins are free, and the first suture is placed as a big bite into the apex of the defect. A continuous suture is ideal, taking good bites of bladder, mucosa and muscle, close together. If a gap is shown later by a dye test, it may be impossible to insert any more sutures. A secure closure is easier with a continuous suture than with an interrupted one. Each suture should be locked. A 5/8-circle needle is perfect in this situation – the tip of the needle is much easier to see and pick up.

Intra-cervical fistulae

Two cases of intra-cervical fistulae are shown in Figures 6.49 and 6.50. A fistula will not be seen in the vagina, and a dye test shows a leak coming through the cervix. These fistulae always result from a caesarean section; most are iatrogenic due to accidental incorporation of some bladder when closing the lower segment. Provided

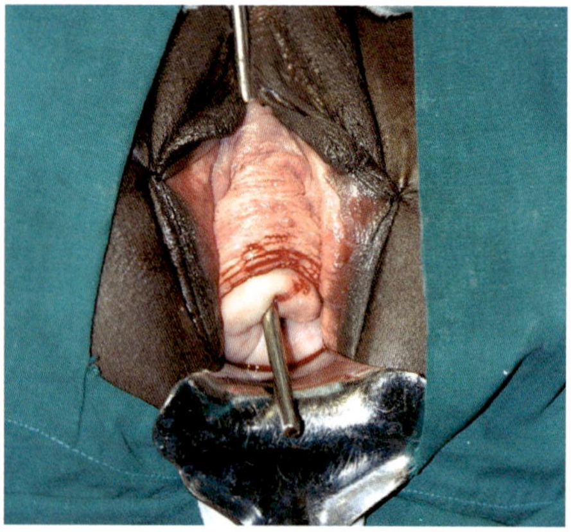

Figure 6.49 In this multiparous patient, the intra-cervical fistula is easily exposed.

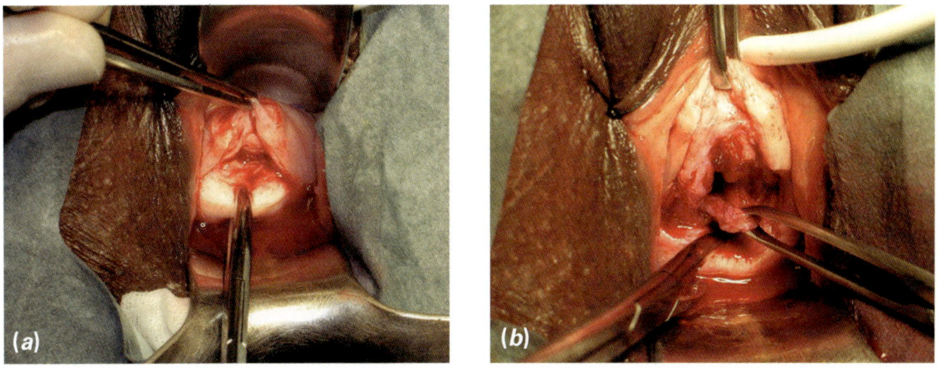

Figure 6.50 (*a*) In this patient, the space between the bladder and anterior cervix has been developed. (*b*) The defect in the bladder can now be seen, and is ready for suture. The ureters could not be found on the fistula margins, and were assumed to be safely distal to the defect.

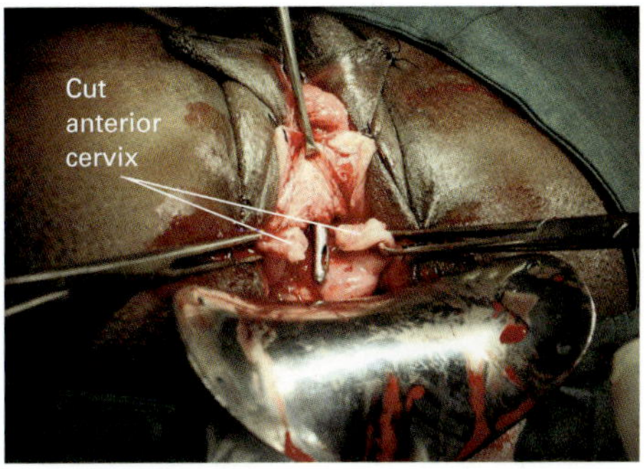

Figure 6.51 The anterior cervix has been cut through to expose the fistula. Strong downward traction on the two sides of the cervix will aid dissection of the bladder to expose the top of the fistula.

that the cervix comes down well, they are not difficult to repair from below (as in the case shown in Figures 6.49 and 6.50).

In some cases, I have found it helpful to cut vertically through the anterior cervix, with the metal catheter passing through the fistula (Figure 6.51). Strong traction on the cut margins of the cervix will bring the bladder defect into view, and it will be easier to dissect the adherent bladder beyond the defect to obtain safe closure. The hole will be well above the ureters.

Andrew Browning repairs all intra-cervical fistulae from below, but I elect to repair about one-third of those that I see via an abdominal trans-vesical approach. Those with less experience of vaginal surgery may find it easier to repair all true intra-cervical fistulae from above, although we advise them to learn the vaginal approach as soon as possible. The abdominal approach is described in the next section.

THE ABDOMINAL APPROACH

When is an abdominal repair appropriate?

Several full-time fistula surgeons, including Andrew Browning, claim that they can repair all fistulae by the vaginal route, however high the fistulae might be. With increasing experience, I have found that I can close the majority of high juxta-cervical, intra-cervical or vault fistulae from below.

I do, however, still find some cases extremely difficult to close from below, and in early days had some bad experiences where, having persisted from below, I had been unable to complete the closure. I strongly believe that there are some cases that are much more easily closed electively by the abdominal route. These are always patients who have sustained their fistula after a caesarean delivery.

It should be noted that an abdominal trans-vesical approach is not an easy opt-out for a fistula that an inexperienced surgeon might find difficult from below. It is essential to realize that *any fistula that is below or likely to be close to the ureteric orifices should not be attempted from above*, except by a very experienced surgeon – this approach needs good abdominal relaxation, proper retractors, good light, an ability to catheterize the ureters from inside the bladder and, above all, good suction. These ideal circumstances may not be met in many resource-poor hospitals.

The final decision on approach is usually made on the operating table, with or without an anaesthetic. The factors to consider are the visibility of the fistula and the mobility of the uterus and cervix as assessed on bi-manual examination.

One group that are often easier from above can be selected from the history.

Post-caesarean iatrogenic intra-cervical fistulae

A post-caesarean iatrogenic intra-cervical fistula can be suspected when the patient gives the story that she was delivered of a live baby, and yet is shown to have a leak through the cervix. The fistula is almost always caused by accidental suture of the bladder into the lower uterine segment.

My criteria for an abdominal approach are as follows:

(a) those that are intra-cervical with a cervix that cannot be pulled down easily (this is more likely in primipara than multipara)

(b) post-hysterectomy vault fistulae that will not come down easily.

Before selecting any patient for an abdominal repair, it is essential to be absolutely certain by dye test and vaginal inspection under anaesthesia that the leak is coming through the cervix and not through an occult hole in the vagina. It is quite possible for a small vaginal fistula to coexist with an intracervical or post-ruptured uterus vault fistula.

A trans-vesical repair illustrated: the O'Connor technique of bladder bisection

Most urologists would prefer an extra-peritoneal approach to the bladder. While this has the advantage of minimal disturbance to the abdominal contents, most general/fistula surgeons, myself included, prefer a general laparotomy. This allows much better exposure. I always put a large suture through the fundus of the uterus to use as a retractor (Figure 6.52). Strong traction on this towards the head end greatly helps to bring the adherent bladder and cervix into view.

The adhesions between the bladder and lower segment are dissected a short distance. If the fistula is not soon found, there should be no hesitation about opening the fundus of the bladder, inspecting the interior and splitting the bladder vertically downwards until the fistula is reached and circumscribed (the O'Connor technique) (Figure 6.53). This, of course, has the added advantage of allowing identification and, if necessary, catheterization of the ureteric orifices. The procedure is illustrated further in Figures 6.54 and 6.55.

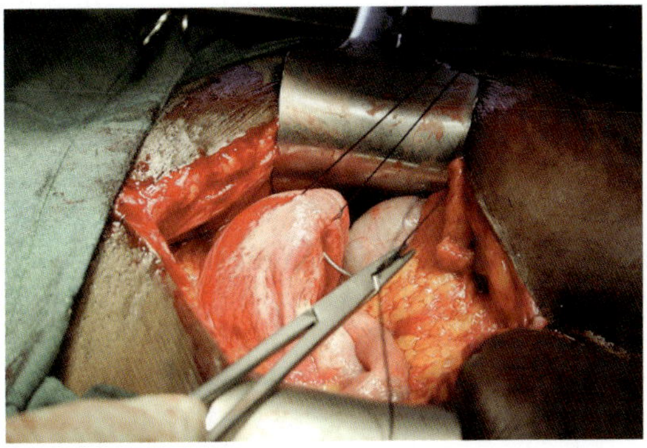

Figure 6.52 A strong suture is placed through the uterine fundus. Strong headward traction makes access to the bladder and fistula much easier.

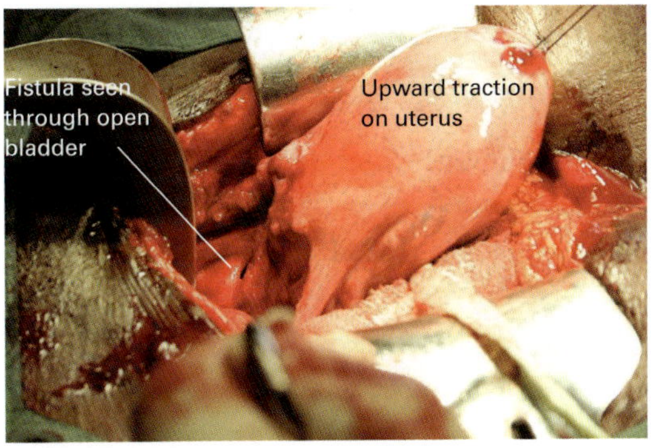

Figure 6.53 An iatrogenic intra-cervical fistula at the level of the old lower segment incision is seen. The bladder has been opened wide through the fundus, and the interior is exposed with a Sims speculum. Note the strong traction applied to the uterus to bring the fistula into view. The ureteric orifices are well below and can easily be demonstrated by giving intravenous furosemide. If at risk, the patient is catheterized.

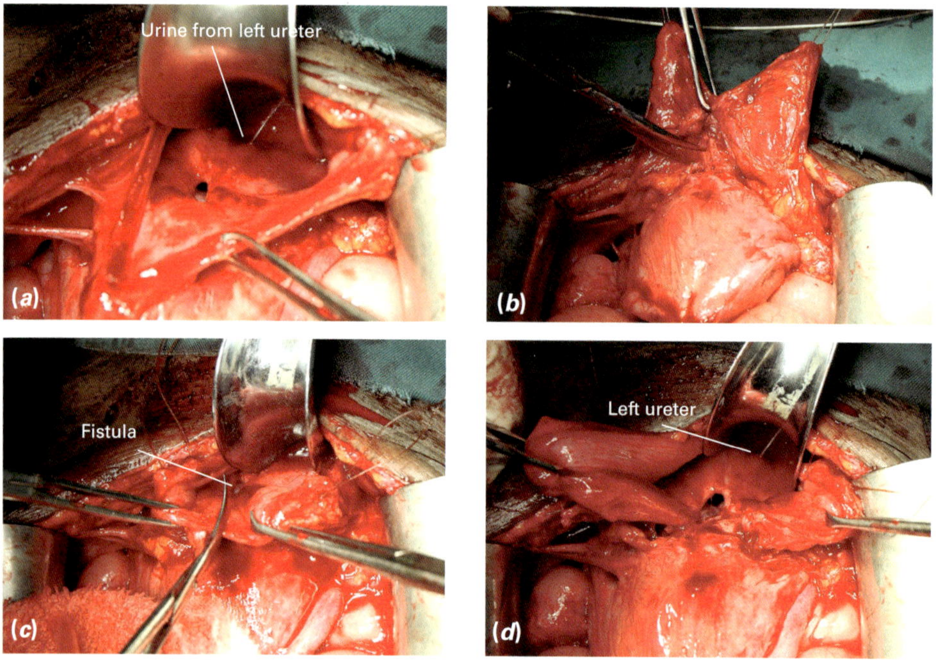

Figure 6.54 (*a*) A view into the opened bladder seen from the head end. There is a post-caesarean fistula between the bladder and an open cervical canal. The bladder has been opened through the vault; on inspecting the interior, the fistula is easily seen and the left ureteric orifice, shown squirting urine, is well below the fistula. Initially, a vaginal approach was considered here, but the distal margin of the fistula could not be seen through the open anterior cervix, so this approach was abandoned. Clearly, it was much easier to close with a trans-vesical approach. (*b*) The bladder is dissected off the lower segment before cutting down into the fistula. (*c*) The bladder is split vertically into the fistula. Strong upward traction on the uterus aids exposure. (*d*) The fistula is opened and the left ureteric orifice is seen well below. The bladder margins will be dissected off the open anterior cervical canal. The cervical defect is closed with two sutures and the bisected bladder is closed with one layer of continuous sutures, beginning with a good bite of bladder at the bottom of the incision. A 5/8-circle needle is ideal. Sutures used to close the cervix should be left long and used to secure a small omental pedicle that will lie behind the bladder repair.

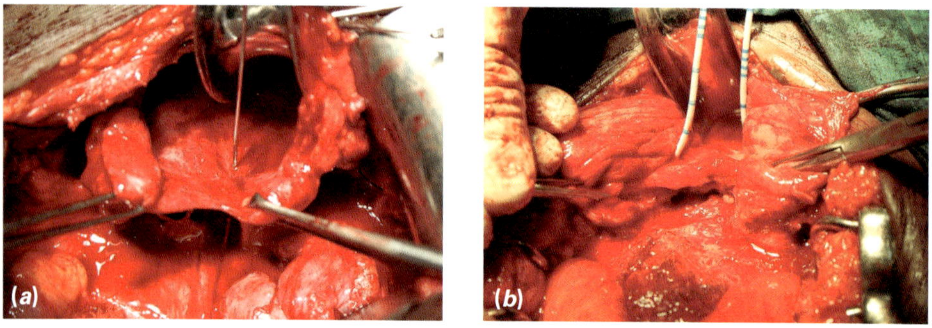

Figure 6.55 (*a, b*) In this example of a post-hysterectomy vault fistula, it has been marked with a probe, and the bladder has then been cut down into it. The ureteric orifices were close, and were catheterized. The fistula has been detached from the vagina, and the bladder is ready for a vertical closure in one layer.

URETHRAL RECONSTRUCTION

About 2% of cases present with complete loss of the urethra. This results from very low obstructed labour in which all the urethra is crushed and sloughs away. It may be a localized injury with a normal-sized bladder, but more commonly occurs with a vesico-vaginal component as well. These defects can be repaired, but it is difficult to achieve a satisfactory functional result. Currently, two methods are available to help restore these patients:

- creation of a new urethra from existing tissue
- construction of a new urethra from the anterior wall of the bladder.

Creation of a new urethra from existing tissue

A new urethra is made from remaining vaginal and para-urethral tissue. However, if all urethral tissue has gone, the prospect is more or less hopeless (Figure 6.56).

If a strip of normal urethral tissue remains, there is a chance of making a reasonable tube. The repair is done by making a U-shaped incision, with the arms of the 'U' extending to where the external urethral meatus should be and about 3 cm apart (Figure 6.57). It is better to make the arms wider than appears necessary, as it is easy to end up with too little tissue to make a tube. The base of the 'U' lies over the

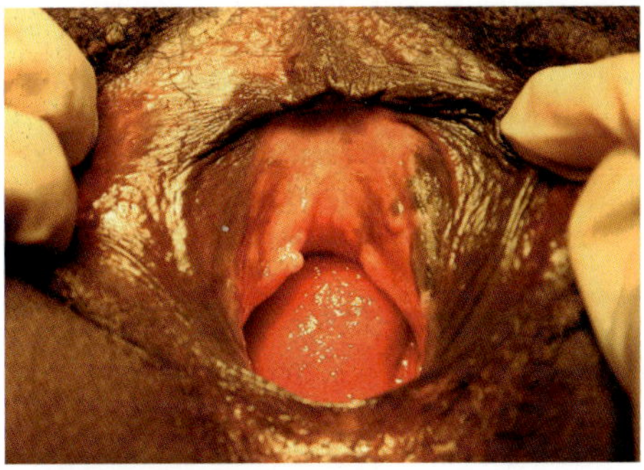

Figure 6.56 Complete destruction of the urethra together with a large vesico-vaginal fistula. The original intention was to make a new urethra out of the anterior bladder wall, but this proved impossible because of the lack of tissue. The patient later had a Mainz pouch.

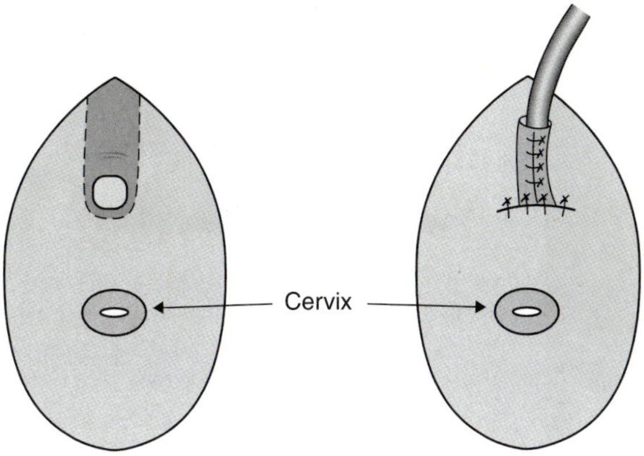

Figure 6.57 Incisions for construction of a new urethra from skin. The gap between the two limbs of the U-shaped incision should be 3 cm.

entrance to the bladder. The sides of the 'U' are undermined a little from either side towards the midline. Care has to be taken, as the tissue is often fragile. The vagina lateral to the U-shaped incision is also dissected to create flaps to cover the new urethra, and the bladder is mobilized as much as necessary to enable it to be attached to the new urethra. The medial flaps are sewn over a Foley catheter. An alternative is to suture the flaps without an indwelling catheter but just to check the diameter of the new urethra after each stitch with a medium Hegar dilator. When completed, a 14 or 16 FG Foley catheter is passed. The catheter must not be tight within the new urethra. The new urethra is then anastomosed to the bladder. We prefer to support the structure with a sling of fibro-muscular tissue from the lateral pelvis, and we sometimes also use a Martius graft as an extra support to the often fragile repair. Occasionally there is insufficient skin either side of the new urethra to cover it. A better alternative is to extend two incisions down the vaginal wall in the direction of the cervix and, having mobilized a flap off the bladder, advance it distally to cover the new urethra.

The results of this operation are not encouraging, with the majority of patients still remaining with urethral incontinence, and later stricture formation is quite common. In effect, it merely makes a tube in which the insertion of a urethral plug might make the patient dry.

The case illustrated in Figure 6.58 shows the principle of repair, and has an excellent prognosis as it is not a childbirth injury. It is a case of traumatic urethral injury from a Gishiri cutting injury in which the superficial urethra has been cut as far as the bladder neck (this is a form of genital mutilation still sometimes practised in Northern Nigeria). As there is no ischaemic tissue loss this is the most favourable type to repair. Figure 6.59 illustrates a case where there is a small bridge of urethra superficially but good urethra on the deep aspect.

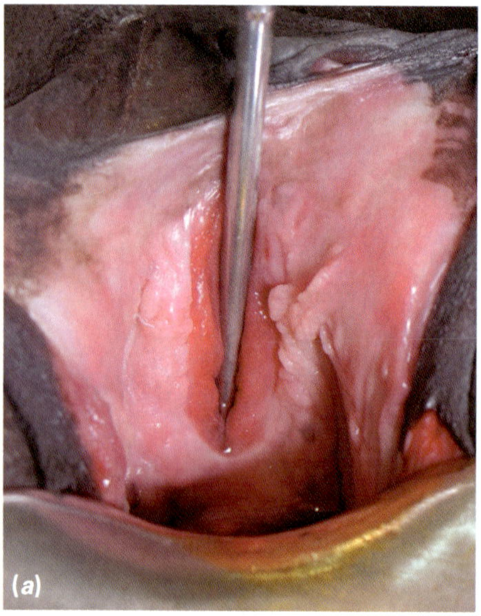

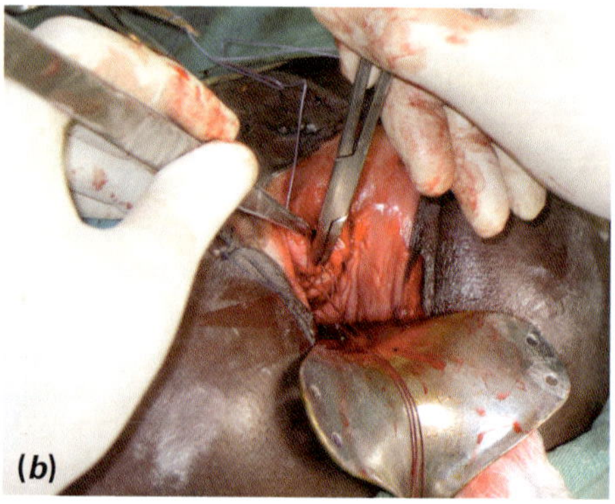

Figure 6.58 (*a*) A metal catheter lies in the wide-open urethra. (*b*) After making the U-shaped incision, the urethra is undermined medially and the vagina laterally. Repair of the urethra is commenced over forceps or a dilator intermittently introduced.

Continued

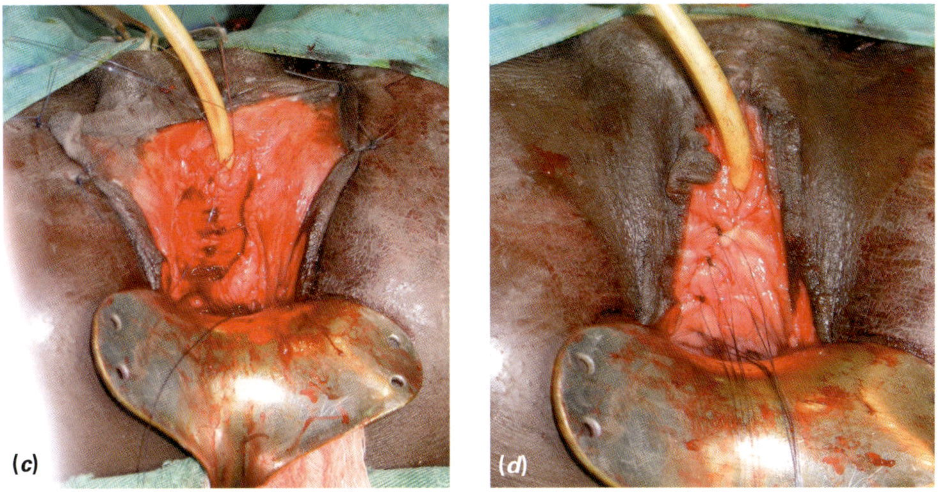

Figure 6.58 (*continued*) (*c*) The urethra has been repaired. (*d*) The mobilized vagina has been closed over the repair. (Photographs taken at Katsina, courtesy of Kees Waaldijk.)

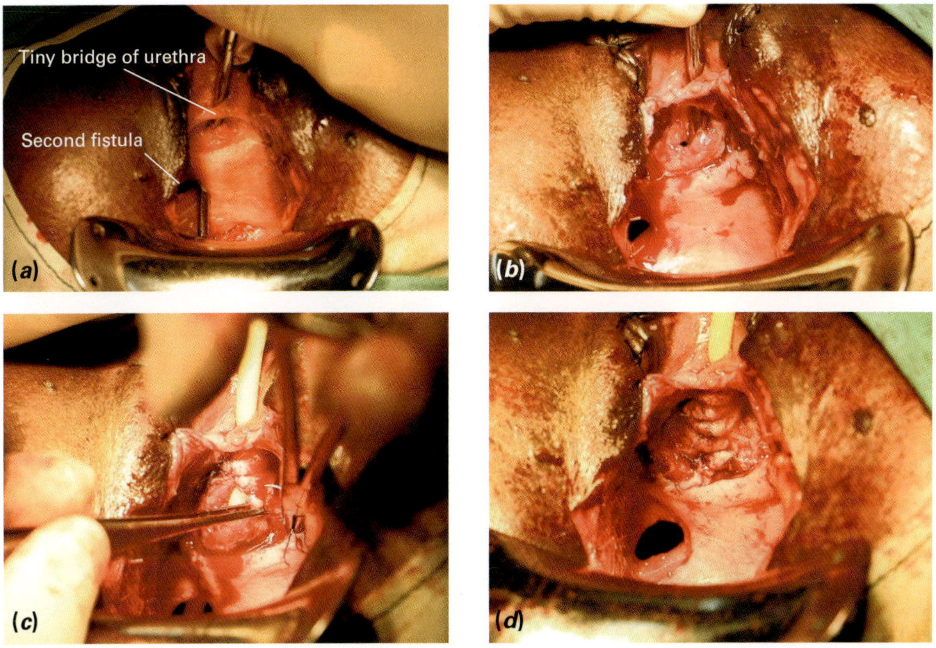

Figure 6.59 (*a*) A tiny bridge of urethra remains. Note a second proximal fistula. (*b*) The para-urethral space has been opened on both sides through a U-shaped incision. (*c*) A new proximal urethra is made over a Foley catheter. (*d*) The repair of the urethral fistula is completed before repairing the second fistula.

Construction of a new urethra from the anterior wall of the bladder

An alternative operation when there is little remaining urethral tissue is to make a new urethra from a flap of anterior bladder wall (Figures 6.60 and 6.61).[4] The results are a little better, and the stricture rates less, but the procedure is technically more difficult and the bladder must be of almost normal size for it to be feasible. This approach is recommended only for advanced fistula surgeons.

For this operation, the bladder has to be mobilized circumferentially and quite widely to bring the anterior wall of the bladder down to where the external urethral meatus should be. When this has been achieved, two incisions are made in the anterior bladder about 3 cm apart and about 2–3 cm long. This flap will become the new urethra. First, the bed of the old urethra over the symphysis pubis needs to have the epithelia removed to create a raw area where the new urethra will lie. The vagina needs to be reflected laterally from where the urethra will lie to cover it later.

The flap is attached in the midline where the external urinary meatus should lie, and is then sewn from side to side over a Foley catheter. A size 12 may be needed if the flap is small. It is sometime easier to attach the bladder to the site of the external meatus before cutting the flap, and then start to sew the bladder from side to side over the catheter, making the incisions in the bladder on proceeding down the length of the urethra. This prevents the serious error of cutting the flap short or narrow.

When the urethra is made over the catheter, the remaining defect in the bladder is repaired either vertically or horizontally, a dye test is performed and a fibro-muscular sling is placed beneath the urethra. A Martius graft is optional.

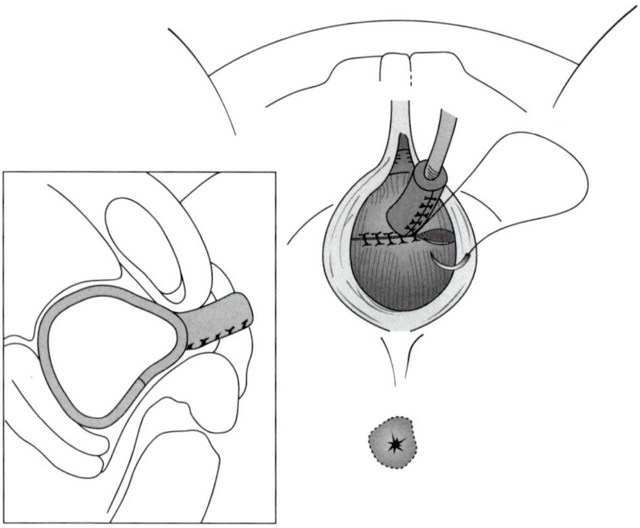

Figure 6.60 Constructing a new urethra from anterior bladder wall.

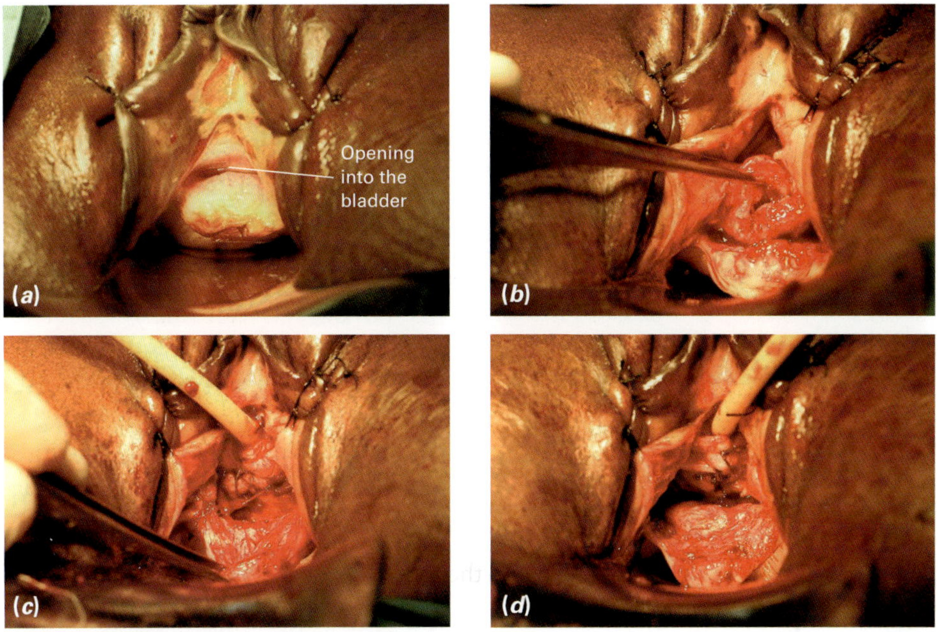

Figure 6.61 (*a*) There is no urethra. (*b*) The bladder is completely mobilized and its anterior wall is held in forceps. Fortunately, there is little loss of bladder tissue. (*c*) A tube made from anterior bladder wall. (*d*) The urethra is supported by a fibro-muscular sling.

Of a small series of ten operations carried out by Andrew Browning, two were completely cured and voiding normally and three had urinary retention but were dry self-catheterizing. The remaining five were still incontinent, although four were able to use a urethral plug and be continent; one was not able to, as her urethra was made too wide and, even with the plug, urine leaked out via the urethra.

This tube of anterior bladder wall can also be used to anastomose to a short urethra. This is technically demanding, and is not often possible because patients who might benefit usually have small bladders, effectively ruling out this step. Browning has used this technique a few times, with modest success.

VAGINAL SKIN DEFECTS

Sometimes, there is no vaginal skin to cover a successful bladder repair. In such cases, there are four options, three of which are simple:

1. Leave it as it is (Figure 6.62).
2. Cover the bladder repair with a fat graft and leave a vaginal defect (Figure 6.63).
3. Use a labial pedicle (Figure 6.64).
4. Use more complicated flaps, e.g. medial thigh or buttock flaps.

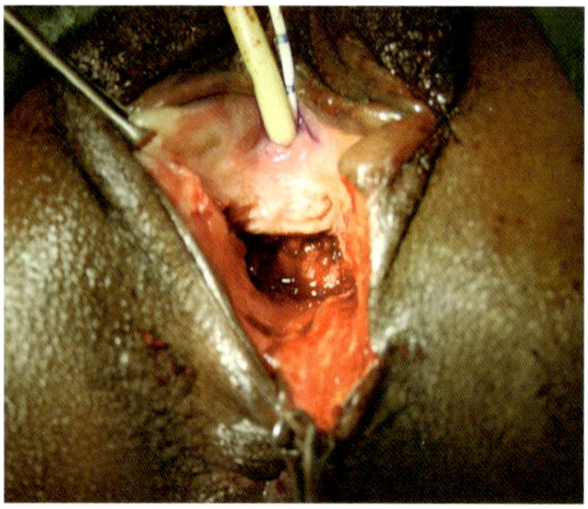

Figure 6.62 A short stenosed vagina with an anterior vaginal defect after repair.

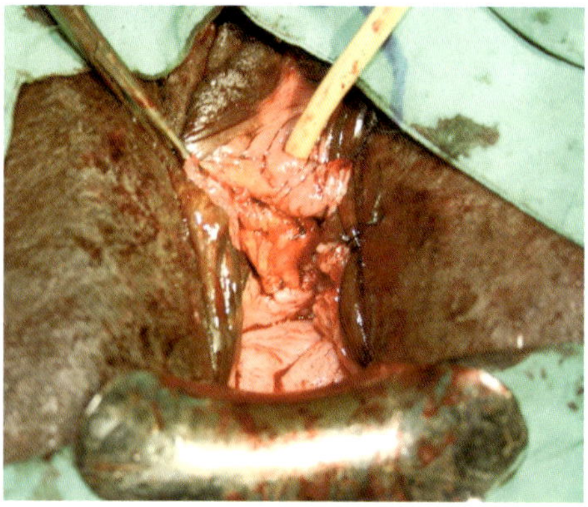

Figure 6.63 This defect is similar to that in Figure 6.62, but has been covered by a fat graft, leaving the vaginal skin to grow over it.

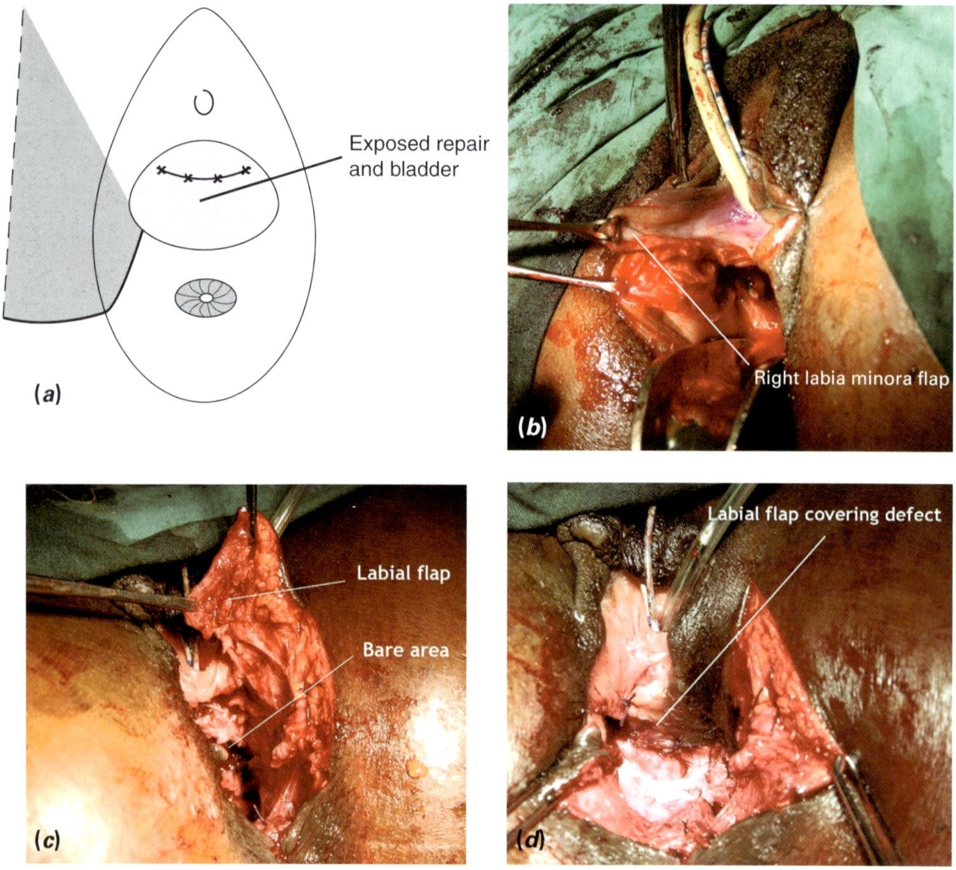

Figure 6.64 (*a*) The labial flap. A vertical incision is made from the existing episiotomy. This can be up the labia majora as for a fat graft or in the grove between labia majora and minora. The shaded area is undermined and rotated as required to cover the defect. (*b*) A flap of labia minora has been raised ready to swing into the defect. (*c*) A labia majora flap is raised. (*d*) The defect is covered.

My present preferred option is to use method 1 or 2. Andrew Browning prefers the third option, usually employing a flap consisting of labia minora.

The cases where this is necessary invariably have significant vaginal stenosis both before and after the repair – the question at stake is whether these different options have any influence on the success of the repair and subsequent continence. We do not know.

If a fat graft is used, a larger skin pedicle can be taken by extending the labial incision down and then into the vagina to meet either the episiotomy incision or the reflection of the vaginal skin that has been made during dissection. An objection to this is that it may bring hair-bearing skin into the vagina. The same objection applies to the apparently attractive option of bringing in an island of labial skin with a fat graft. A better option is just to use labia minora, which do not bear any hair.

Some surgeons use more radical flaps taken from the medial thigh or buttock. The hope is that these will increase vaginal capacity and possibly help in improving closure and continence rates. However, this approach adds to the morbidity of the operation. We have little experience with these flaps, and remain to be convinced of their value.

THE MARTIUS FAT GRAFT

To graft or not to graft?

For 30 years, a Martius fat graft (in reality a pedicle) has been the mainstay of completing a repair for all but the simplest fistulae at the Addis Ababa Fistula Hospital. When introduced, it appeared to result in significantly improved results. However, in recent years, many experienced fistula surgeons have used it less and less, until it has been all but abandoned, without compromising results.

The idea of the Martius fat graft is to bring good tissue with its blood supply into the area of the repair. The graft appears quite vascular, as it is raised from its bed, but, when pulled into the vagina, there is rarely any sign of bleeding; if an old fat graft is found at a re-repair, it shows little sign of vascularity and resembles a lipoma.

Its proponents claimed that it improved closure rates, and still claim that it fills dead space. It has also been suggested that a pad of fat between the bladder and vagina may offer some protection should the patient be forced by circumstances beyond her control into a vaginal delivery again.

The downside of a fat graft is the extra time and extra use of sutures and the slight increased risk of a haematoma.

We rarely use fat grafts. Our possible indications are:

- Sometimes to cover a repair where there is lack of vaginal skin.

- As a last-ditch attempt to close a defect that has failed several times. We know of two cases successfully closed at a fifth attempt using a fat graft on the last repair. (Both repairs had been performed on the last occasion by a very experienced surgeon, which could be the reason for the success.)
- On those few occasions where it has been impossible to achieve a watertight closure.
- To support a urethral repair.

As there may still be a place for the use of the Martius fat graft in selected cases, a description will be given here. We currently use a graft in about 1 in 50 repairs.

The Martius graft

After completing the bladder repair, five anchor sutures are placed (Figure 6.65):

- Two sutures above the fistula – one on each side, high and laterally, usually using the corner sutures (1 and 2), which have been left long.
- Three sutures proximal to the repair – two in the side wall of the vagina (3 and 4) and one on the midline (5) either into the cervix, if the dissection has extended this far, or at the top of the reflected vaginal wall.

Note that anchor sutures are not put in the bladder. The sutures are left long, and will be threaded onto eyed needles to pass through the graft.

The operating table is taken out of the Trendelenburg position to bring the labia into comfortable view. The right labia is traditionally used. The sutures that were used to retract the distal vaginal skin on this side are cut.

The landmark for the incision is on the most prominent bulge of the labia majora beginning lateral to the base of the clitoris, down the prominence of the labia for at least 6 cm. It helps to make a clean incision if these landmarks are grasped with the stronger Littlewoods tissue forceps and tension is applied between these points (Figure 6.66a).

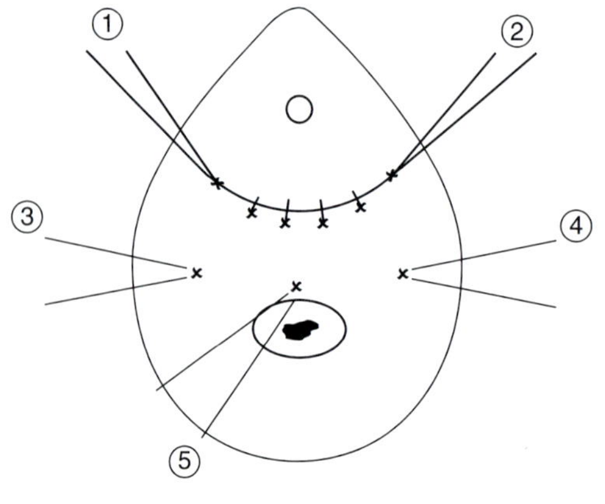

Figure 6.65 Placement of five anchor sutures in preparation for a Martius fat graft.

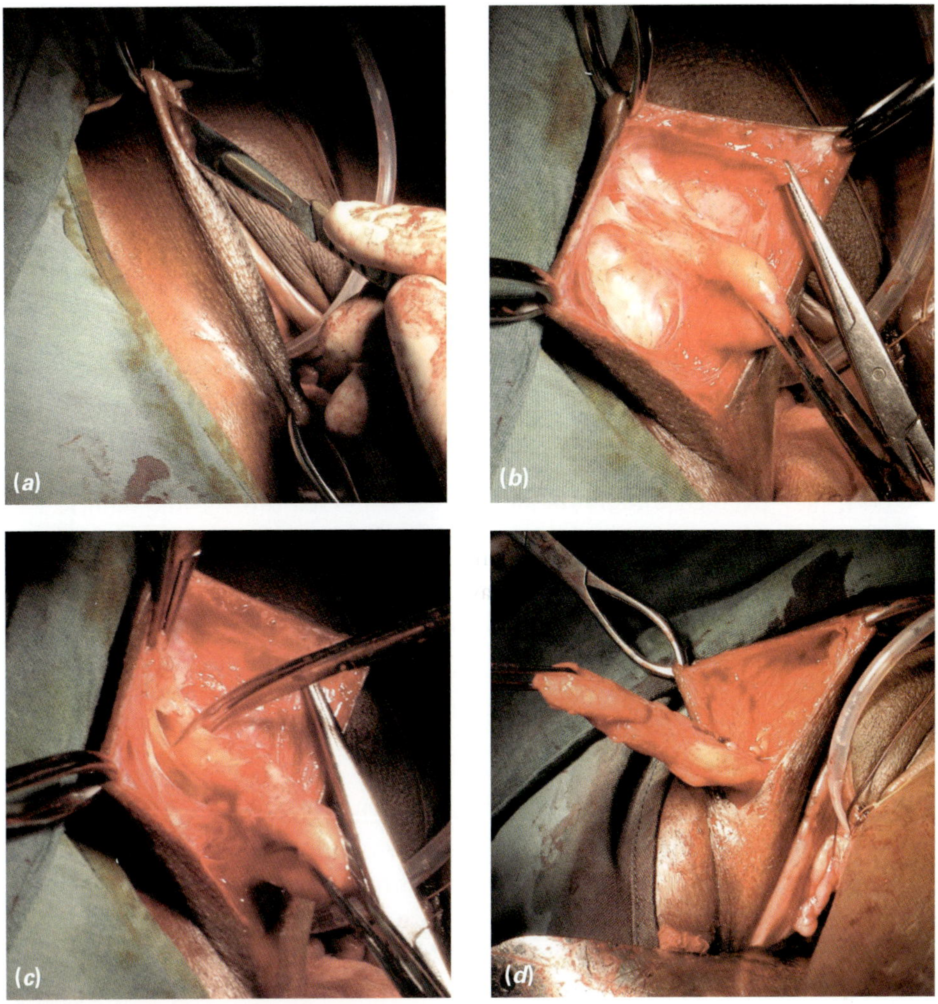

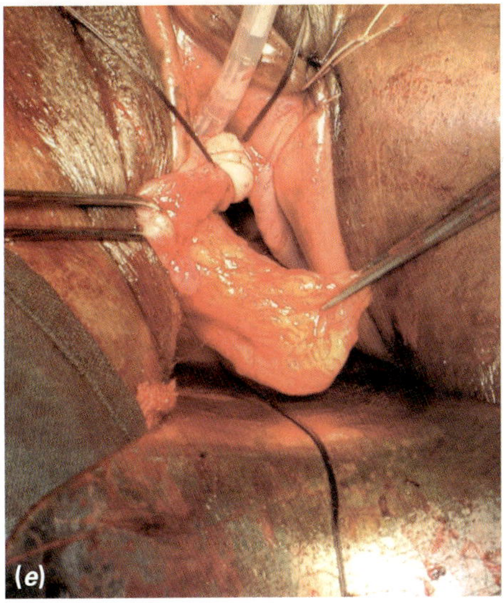

Figure 6.66 Martius fat graft. (*a*) Skin incision between Littlewoods forceps. (*b*) The fat pad is grasped with Allis forceps. (*c*) The pedicle is dissected off the underlying deep fascia. (*d*) The completed pedicle. (*e*) The fat has been pulled into the vagina.

The skin and subcutaneous tissue are incised and the fat pad beneath is exposed. The fat pad is grasped with an Allis forceps (Figure 6.66b), and reflected off the underlying skin laterally and medially. This is area is vascular, especially its medial edge, so attention must be paid to securing haemostasis.

The pedicle of fat is cut level with the top of the incision and dissected downwards off the underlying deep fascia (Figure 6.66c). The dissection continues until the medial margin of the inferior pubic ramus is reached and a tunnel can be formed into the vagina. The raised pedicle is attached inferiorly to maintain its blood supply (Figure 6.66d).

Haemostasis is obtained and then the graft is introduced into the vagina by making a tunnel with the dissecting scissors between the labia and the inferior pubic ramus. It may be necessary to extend the vaginal incision further distally. The vaginal flap is lifted up. The scissors are introduced and the blades are opened a little to enlarge the hole; they are then withdrawn and a finger is pushed through the tunnel. The tunnel must be large enough to accommodate the fat pedicle so that it will not strangulate.

The fat pedicle is introduced into the vagina through this tunnel with the aid of an Allis forceps and is sutured into place using the five anchor sutures placed previously (Figure 6.66e). The free ends of the sutures are threaded onto a blank needle and both are brought through the fat and tied. The graft should be spread out and lie neatly over the whole of the repair.

The graft site on the labia must be repaired carefully. The area is prone to haematoma formation. The closure is done is three layers, beginning superiorly by taking a large bite with a 0 chromic or Vicryl suture through the previously cut labial fat. The suture is taken continuously down and then back up, closing all potential dead space. The final layer is of interrupted skin sutures.

BLADDER STONES

Bladder calculi are found in only about 2% of new cases, but their correct management is very important.

Causes

Bladder stones may be caused by:

- foreign material pushed up the vagina into the bladder in an attempt to stop the leak
- crystals forming in concentrated urine and growing over time
- non-absorbable sutures used in bladder repair (e.g. damage during caesarean section) (Figure 6.67).

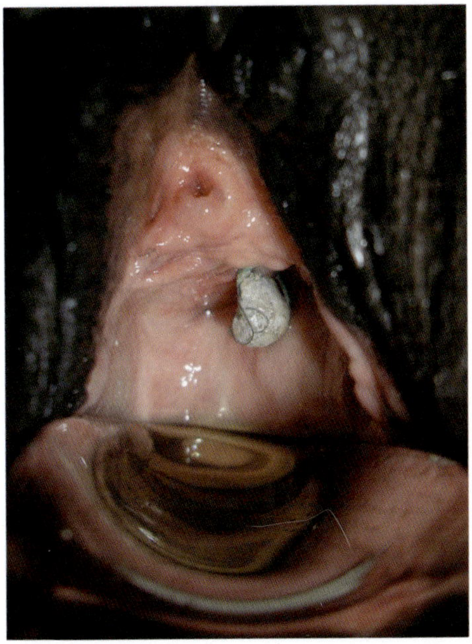

Figure 6.67 This residual fistula has a stone around a non-absorbable suture that was mistakenly used in the repair.

Detection

Bladder calculi almost always occur with small fistulae, although exceptionally a large calculus may be found half in, half out of a large fistula.

Bladder calculi may cause an enormous amount of discomfort, and can often be suspected preoperatively when there is tenderness on vaginal examination. A complaint or an observation of haematuria is another sign. The urine is usually infected and smelly.

A large stone can be felt on gentle bimanual examination, and any stone can be detected by sounding inside the bladder with a metal probe (Figure 6.68).

Small stones may be missed on clinical assessment. It is vital to detect and remove all stones before embarking on a repair. A missed stone is a disaster. We have seen patients return some time after a successful repair in great distress from a large stone. It is probable that a small one was missed at the repair.

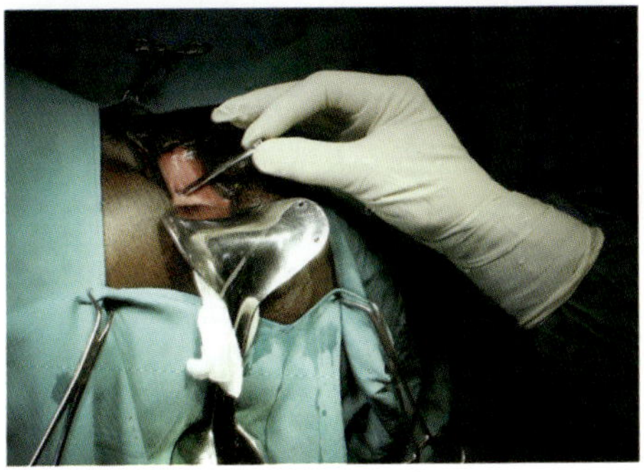

Figure 6.68 Sounding for bladder stones.

Management

Repair of a fistula should be delayed until after removal of a stone. In the presence of a stone, the bladder is thick-walled and hyperaemic, and there is almost certainly urinary infection. These conditions are not conducive for a successful repair. The interval between removal and safe repair may only be about 2 weeks, but each case should be assessed on its merits and local circumstances.

We prefer to remove stones by a suprapubic extra-peritoneal approach (Figure 6.69).

Exceptionally, the stone may protrude though the fistula into the vagina, and it may be easy to remove it this way without having to enlarge the fistula too much (Figure 6.70). To remove most calculi through the vagina would require an enormous enlargement of the fistula that does not seem justified.

Infection is usual, and it is essential to give perioperative antibiotic cover. We use intravenous gentamicin 160 mg for the operation, followed by 80 mg, 8-hourly for 48 hours. Exceptionally, septicaemia has occurred after stone extraction.

Exposure should be through a generous lower midline incision, with a large cut into the bladder to extract the stone with sponge forceps. It is useful have an assistant exerting upward pressure from the vagina. Fortunately, most stones are solitary and firm, and do not crumble on extraction. If the stone does break into fragments, it is vital that they all be washed out and removed. Even one small residue will lead to another stone.

The bladder can be closed and drained through a urethral catheter, although we usually prefer to close the bladder loosely around a suprapubic catheter. The urethra is often gaping in patients with calculi, so it may be best to rest the urethra in the pre-repair period.

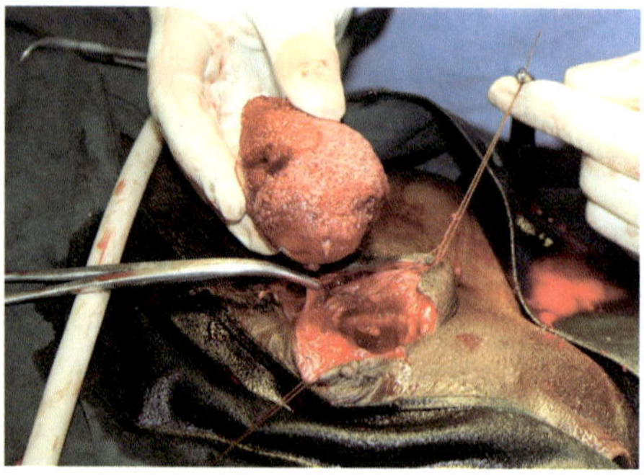

Figure 6.69 A large stone removed by suprapubic incision.

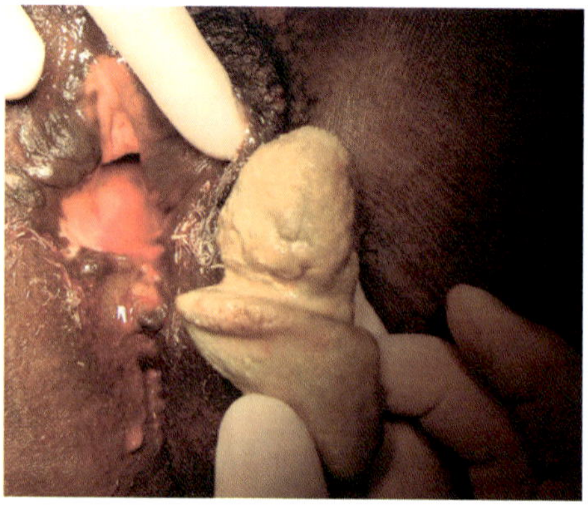

Figure 6.70 This stone was protruding into the vagina, and was removed easily. Note the waist indicating the fistula margins. The fistula was successfully repaired 2 weeks later.

FAILED REPAIR AND RE-OPERATION

Breakdown of a repair is a major disappointment. It may be because the operation was not done well, because of neglectful postoperative care (catheter blockage) or occasionally because of postoperative infection. The usual reason for failure is that the damage was so severe as to preclude an adequate repair. Identifiable risk factors for breakdown are previous operation, severe scarring, destruction of the urethra, a small bladder, ureteric orifices outside the bladder and concurrent recto-vaginal fistula.

We find that about 15% of new patients presenting to us have had a previous repair elsewhere. Many of these cases are still quite easy to cure, as they were simple ones inexpertly done, but of course we also have to operate on some of our own failures.

The rare occurrence of wetness on the day following a repair deserves a dye test in theatre. The most likely explanation is the presence of an overlooked ureteric fistula as well as the vesico-vaginal fistula. If this is confirmed, a ureteric implant can be performed electively in the postoperative period. This has occurred four times in my series. If, however, the dye test is positive and the repair was thought to be sound, it is tempting to take the patient back to try and stop the leak with additional sutures. Provided that the re-operation is performed within 48 hours, the bladder will hold additional sutures well, and, on the two occasions when this has been tried, the leak was stopped. After 48 hours, the tissues become oedematous and further suturing is unlikely to be successful. Breakdowns occurring in the second or third week after repair have a better prognosis, and some will close with prolonged bladder drainage. Their management is described in Chapter 11.

The principles of a re-repair are no different to those for a new case. There will, however, be less healthy tissue available, more scar and distorted anatomy. This is particularly so when a repair has been attempted by an inexperienced surgeon. Clearly, the patient needs to be carefully assessed prior to the operation, noting the presence of any of the risk factors, and the surgeon needs to decide if he or she is confident enough to operate. We advise waiting at least 3 months before attempting a re-repair.

A few breakdowns will be in the middle of the old repair and therefore easily accessible, but the majority are small and inaccessible at the lateral margins of the repair or at the corners of a circumferential anastomosis (Figure 6.71). There are a number of tips for repairing these. First, exposure must be optimal, with episiotomies if necessary. Small corner defects that are are high in the anterior vaginal fornix can often be approached directly, but better access may be obtained by mobilizing the bladder off the cervix and advancing up the side wall of the bladder to the defect. Elevation of the vaginal skin off the defect is greatly helped by Thorek scissors. It is impossible to find the ureteric orifice through small holes, and we simply close the defect with two or three sutures. As the lateral margin is often close to bone, it is important to take strong bites and the insert all the sutures before tying them. A small J or 5/8-circle needle is a great help here. Wherever possible, we swing a small flap of fibro-muscular tissue from under the pubic arch as a reinforcement.

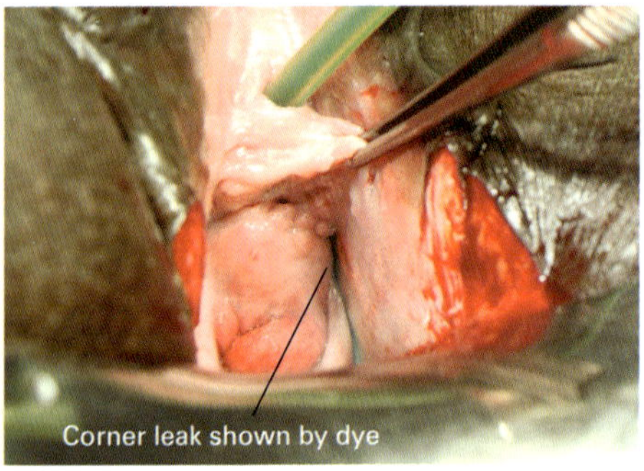

Figure 6.71 A dye test has shown a small leak from the corner of a previous repair. Note that the anterior vaginal wall is very short. The cervix is close to the old repair site.

In the case of slightly larger defects, we rarely enlarge them to see inside the bladder, but just check that the ureteric orifice it is not on the margin of the defect by probing or with the help of intravenous furosemide. Using this minimalist approach, we have not knowingly had any problems with ligated ureters.

Residual fistulae high in the region of the cervix following a failed intra-cervical repair provide a special challenge that depends largely on how much the cervix can be pulled down. I have recently had two patients both of whom had two failures by the vaginal approach. They were quite easily cured on their third operation through a trans-vesical approach.

Figures 6.72–6.74 show some examples of re-repairs.

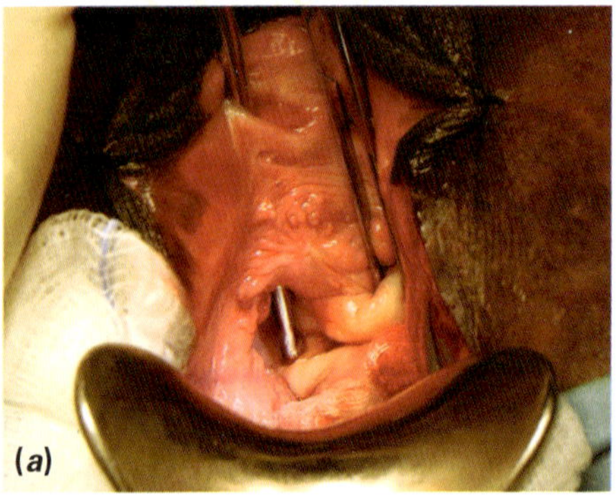

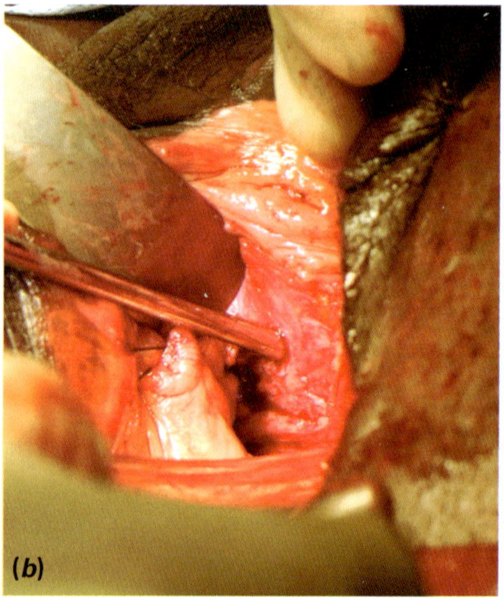

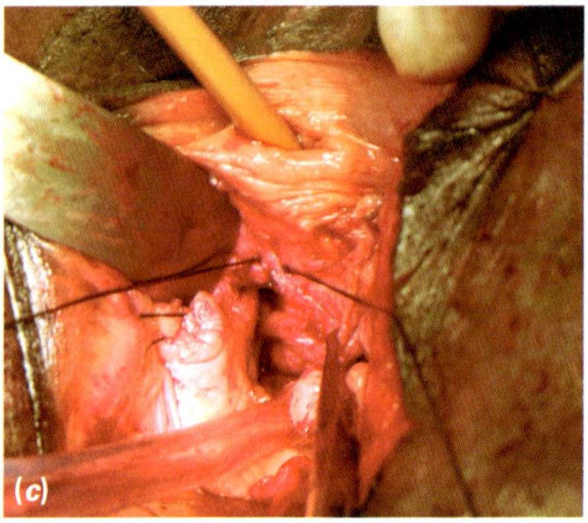

Figure 6.72 (*a*) A high corner residual fistula. (*b*) The space between the cervix and bladder has been opened and the small defect exposed, as indicated by the metal catheter. (*c*) This defect will be closed by two sutures. The first has been inserted.

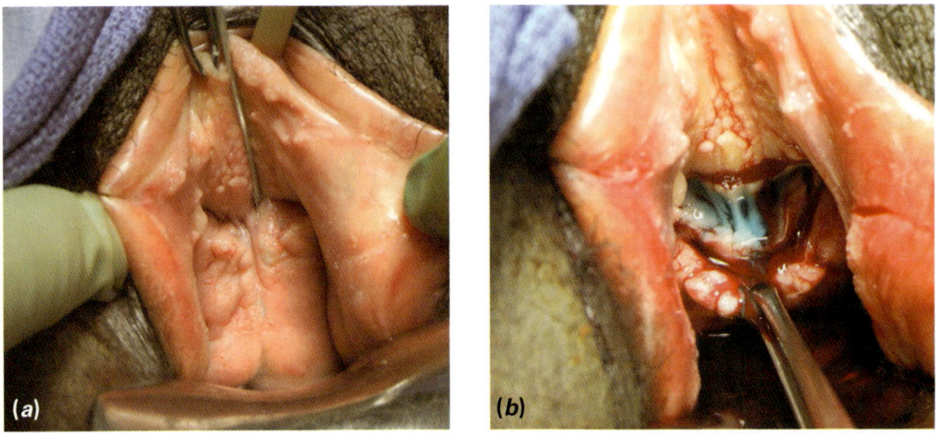

Figure 6.73 (*a*) Multiple residual holes can be seen at an old repair site. (*b*) A dye test showed multiple leaks. The whole area is re-excised, followed by adequate mobilization and repair.

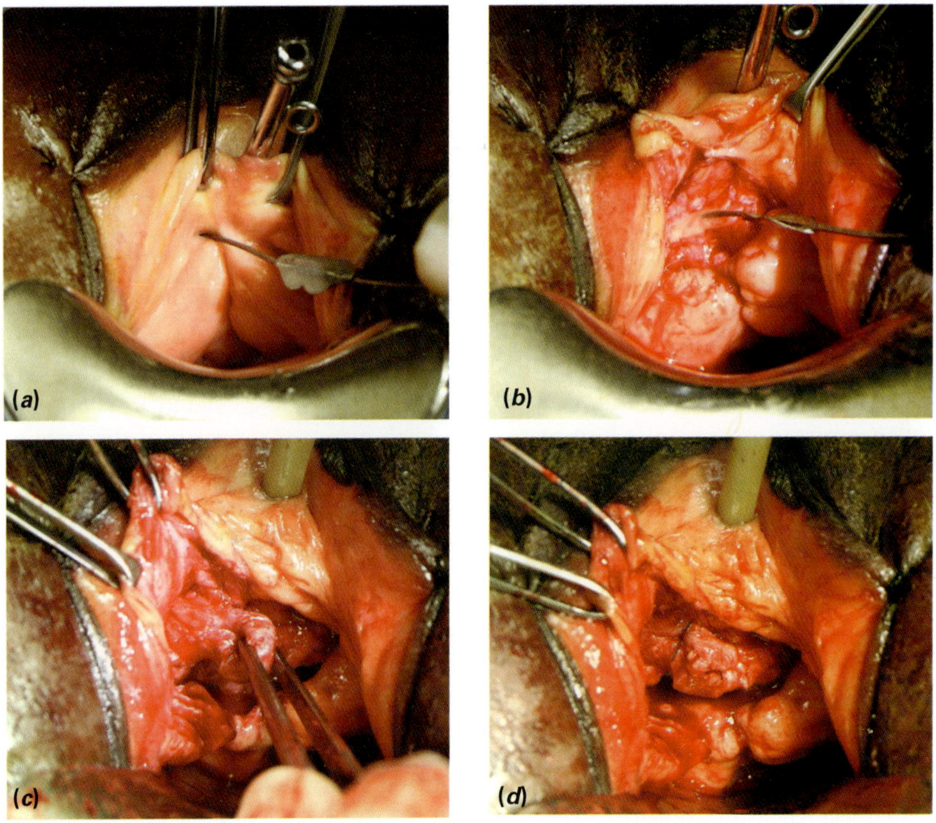

Figure 6.74 (*a*) A tiny accessible corner breakdown. (*b*) The probe is kept in place while the surrounding vagina is elevated. The margins are excised and inverted with two sutures. (*c–d*) A flap of fibro-muscular tissue has been raised (as for a fibro-muscular sling), and is sutured over the repair.

How many times can one go on attempting a repair?

The chance of successful repair diminishes with each attempt, but, as long as there is some reasonable tissue and enough bladder and urethra to function, it is worth going on. We have occasionally seen a repair succeed after up to five attempts. In many patients, however, it will unfortunately be obvious from the degree of scarring, size of bladder and poor urethra that multiple attempts are not appropriate.

Does HIV status affect success?

This is a big unanswered question. Clearly, it would not be sensible to operate on someone who was sick with AIDS, but one sometimes wonders if an unexpected breakdown might be due to a reduced immune status. I have had four patients who had repeated unexplained breakdowns after relatively simple repairs. Two were HIV positive and two were not. To further our understanding of this problem, we do recommend HIV testing with consent for repeated unexpected breakdown. At present, we do not let our knowledge of HIV status influence our decision to operate if other conditions are right.

Results of re-repair

Our results for re-repairs in Uganda and Ethiopia are similar. About 60% of cases with a first time re-repair go home dry. With each successive repair, the results become worse.

URETERIC FISTULAE

Iatrogenic injuries to the ureter are unfortunately quite common. In Uganda, they account for 5% of patients with urinary incontinence following childbirth. About half follow a caesarean section; a history of a live birth increases suspicion of this type of injury. Most commonly, the ureter is caught up while stitching the corners of the lower segment. In some cases, there is silent atrophy of the kidney; in others, the ureter may slough and urine can escape into the cervical canal through the lower-segment incision.

Other cases of ureteric fistula occur after emergency hysterectomy for a ruptured uterus. Considering the difficult conditions and the inexperience of many doctors called upon to treat a ruptured uterus in rural areas, these injuries are understandable. Any urine leaking into the pelvis will soon find its way out between the sutured vaginal vault and cervical remnant.

The third cause of ureteric fistula is unrecognized injury to a ureter at the time of a vesico-vaginal fistula repair. In this situation, it may be possible at a later date to catheterize the ureter and implant it into the bladder transvaginally.

If the patient has several living children, and an abdominal operation is planned, the option of tubal ligation should be discussed. It is easy to do this at the same time as the fistula repair.

Diagnosis of ureteric fistula is discussed in Chapter 2. An ultrasound scan showing a distended ureter on one side is helpful confirmation. However, it is essential to confirm again on the table that the dye test is really negative and that urine appears in the vagina after giving furosemide. In partial injuries, the leak can be very small.

The affected ureter must be identified in the pelvic side wall and traced down to the point of injury. Four times out of five the affected ureter is found to be dilated, and thickening can usually be felt at the site of injury. If the ureter is draining very freely into the vagina, it will not be dilated. The most reliable method of confirming the site of injury is to open the bladder and look inside at the ureteric orifices. Intravenous furosemide 20 mg should be given and the non-functioning side identified. Exceptionally, a partial ureteric injury (e.g. after a previous repair) may still produce urine into the bladder – but not nearly so much as the uninjured side.

If the diagnosis and side of the fistula are certain, some surgeons prefer an extraperitoneal approach, but I prefer a midline incision. The abdominal approach is usually quite easy, and the results are uniformly successful.

In my 44 cases, I have never had a problem making the ureter reach the bladder. The ureter must be divided as low down as possible, and it helps to mobilize the contralateral side of the bladder. If the ureter will not reach the bladder, the possibilities are, in order of preference:

1. Fully mobilize the contralateral side of the bladder and support the anastomosis with a psoas hitch stitch.
2. Make a tube out of the dome of the bladder (Boari's flap).
3. Anastomose the cut ureter end to side to the uninjured ureter.

The steps of the operation are shown in Figure 6.75. I do not splint or drain the anastomosis as a routine when the ureter comes into the bladder without tension. If

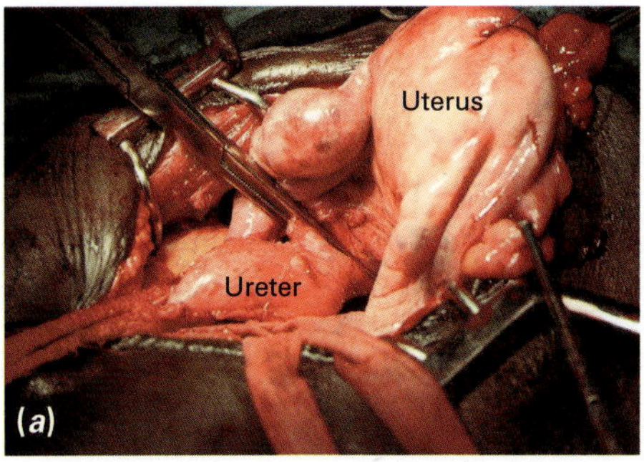

Figure 6.75 (*a*) A very dilated ureter has been clamped at the level of the cervix.

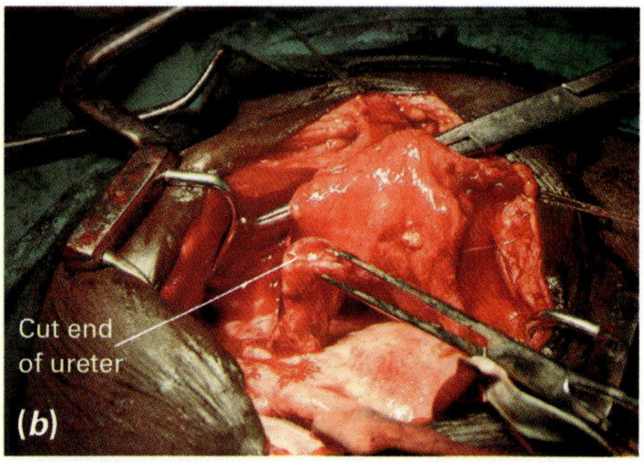

Figure 6.75 (*b*) The bladder has been opened through the fundus and forceps have been pushed through the lateral bladder wall ready to grasp the cut ureter.

Continued

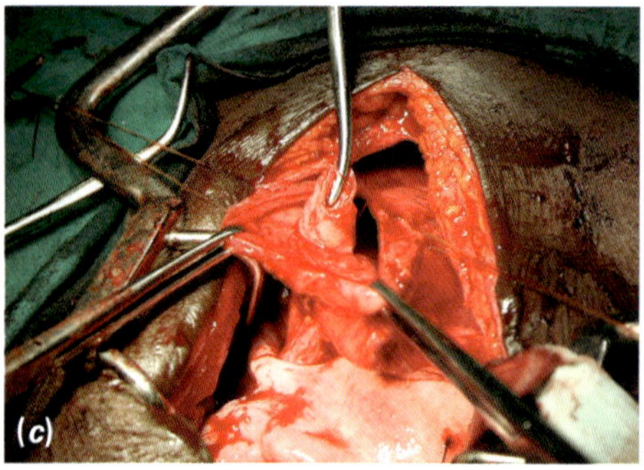

Figure 6.75 (*c*) The ureter is pulled into the bladder.

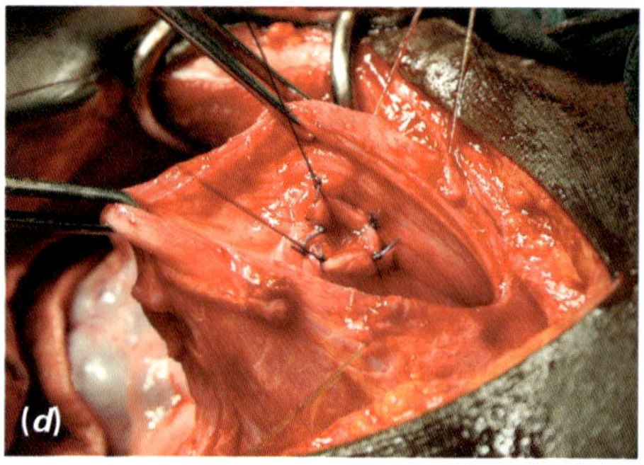

Figure 6.75 (*d*) The ureter is sutured to the bladder mucosa. If not very dilated, it should be spatulated slightly. The sutures just pick up the underlying bladder muscle.

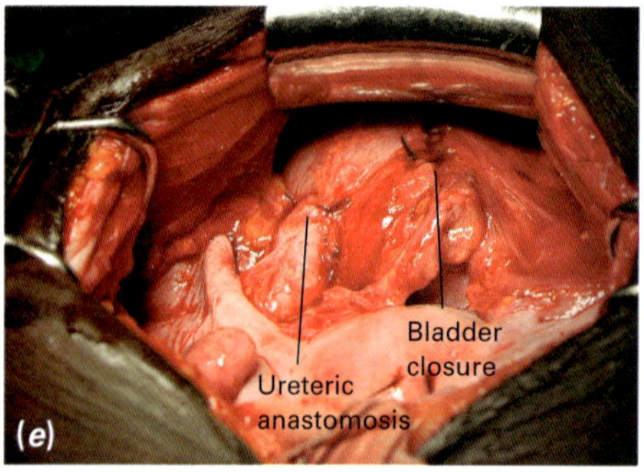

Figure 6.75 (*e*) The adventitia of the ureter is sutured to the bladder muscle with a few interrupted sutures on the outside, and the bladder incision is closed.

in doubt, I would advise that a ureteric catheter be passed through the anastomosis. It will decompress the ureter should there be any hold-up at the anastomosis. The distal end can be brought out alongside a urethral catheter or through a separate stab incision in the anterior bladder wall. The ureteric catheter, if used, can be removed on day 7 and the urinary catheter removed on day 10.

References

1. Browning A. The circumferential obstetric fistula: characteristics, management and outcomes. *Br J Obstet Gynaecol* 2007; **114**: 1172–6.
2. Browning A. Risk factors for developing residual urinary incontinence after obstetric fistula repair. *Br J Obstet Gynaecol* 2006; **113**: 482–5.
3. Browning A. Prevention of residual urinary incontinence following successful repair of obstetric vesico-vaginal fistula using a fibro-muscular sling. *Br J Obstet Gynaecol* 2004; **111**: 357–61.
4. Elkins TE, Ghosh TS, Tagoe GA. Stocker R. Transvaginal mobilization and utilization of the anterior bladder wall to repair vesicovaginal fistulae involving the urethra. *Obstet Gynecol* 1992; **79**: 455–60.

7 Recto-vaginal Fistulae

A recto-vaginal fistula (RVF) is produced only in the most prolonged episodes of obstruction, and so is usually associated with a severe vesico-vaginal fistula (VVF) and neurological damage. Isolated RVFs due to obstructed labour are extremely rare, but may be caused by sexual violence in war situations or in under-age marriage.

Anal sphincter tears usually occur in isolation unrelated to obstructed labour, and should not be classified as RVFs unless there is significant extension into the rectum.

Incompletely repaired sphincter tears are another source of low RVF.

Incidence

The exact incidence of RVF is difficult to determine, because some surgeons classify sphincter injuries as RVFs, where strictly the term should be reserved for a recto-vaginal communication above the level of the sphincter. However, a few injuries do involve the lower rectum and sphincter complex to some extent. Also, if surgeons have been selective in avoiding the most difficult VVFs, the excluded cases will have a higher incidence of RVF, and so the true incidence will be underestimated.

The highest incidence is reported from the Addis Ababa Fistula Hospital, where 15% of VVF patients operated upon have an RVF as well.[1] An unusual incidence of isolated traumatic RVF in under-age brides has been reported from Ethiopia.[2] In Bahr Dar, northern Ethiopia, the incidence of combined fistulae is 8.4%. The figure for Uganda is lower, at 3.3%. The difference between Ethiopia and Uganda can be partly explained by the much lower incidence of caesarean section in the Ethiopian fistula patients (15% vs 65%)

Those patients who eventually deliver vaginally suffer more ischaemia than those whose obstruction is relieved by caesarean section. Thus, the incidence of RVF in those delivered by caesarean section is similar in the two countries at about 2%, whereas for those delivering vaginally, the percentage increases to 5.2% in Uganda but is still significantly below that in Ethiopia at 9.3% ($p = 0.001$).

Classification

An objective classification of RVFs is based on the distance from the site of the hymen to the distal margin of the fistula, as described by Judith Goh.[3] In practice, most people describe RVFs as low, high or intermediate. An estimate is made of the size and the amount of scar surrounding the defect.

Assessment

It is important to recognize that scarring will distort the anatomy of the rectum. A careful assessment by rectal examination is just as important as a vaginal assessment, paying attention to the site, size and degree of scarring. It is common for a fistula felt in the mid-vagina to feel higher than expected on rectal examination. If there is difficulty, a probe should be passed though the vaginal opening to feel where it comes into the rectum. What appears to be a small hole on digital examination may be found at operation to involve almost half the circumference of the rectum. The lumen of the rectum at the level of the fistula must be carefully assessed. Narrowing may well be present, and this will influence the method of closure so as not to occlude the lumen. Exceptionally, the rectum is completely blocked just distal to the fistula (Figure 7.1).

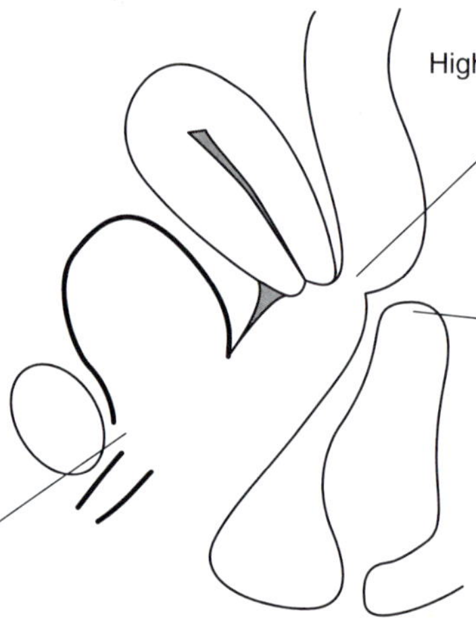

Figure 7.1 A completely stenosed rectum.

The status of the anal sphincter should be recorded. The resting tone, the squeeze pressure and the quality of the pubo-rectalis sling should be estimated.

Does every RVF need to be closed?

Not all RVFs need to be closed. The symptoms of RVF vary from complete faecal incontinence to none. It is often surprising that some patients with a moderate-sized RVF report very little leakage unless they have diarrhoea. Some with tiny fistulae may deny any symptoms at all. There is no point embarking on a potentially difficult repair if the patient has few symptoms.

In spite of every care, a small RVF may be discovered unexpectedly while repairing a bladder fistula by the appearance of bubbles from the rectum. If the RVF is easily accessible, it can be repaired after the VVF, but, if it is high and potentially difficult, it can be safely ignored. I have on four occasions not closed a small RVF after repairing the VVF. This did not compromise the bladder repair.

The discovery of a larger RVF during an operation is an embarrassing error of preoperative assessment, and its management depends on its site and size and the experience of the operator.

Which rectal fistulae require a colostomy?

We believe that colostomies are used far too often for RVFs – a decision about a colostomy should be made only by the surgeon who is going to do the repair, and are rarely required. A colostomy should never be performed by a general surgeon in the vague hope that someone can be found to repair the fistula later. To live with a colostomy is probably of equal misery for the patient as the rectal fistula. We have seen far too many badly made colostomies that have prolapsed, adding to the patient's distress.

Provided that the surgeon believes that the fistula can be closed securely with healthy mobile margins, preferably in two layers, and the lower bowel is empty, there is no need for a colostomy.

Experienced surgeons recognize that some RVFs that are high, large and surrounded by scar are going to be very difficult to close securely, and feel happier if a preliminary colostomy has been made. Colostomies are not going to increase the chance of healing – they simply lessen the postoperative complications of sepsis or peritonitis should a major breakdown occur.

A strategy that I have found to work for the high difficult fistula is to do as much as possible of the mobilization trans-vaginally and then to open the abdomen and complete the repair from above. It is then much easier to perform an accurate two-layer closure, for which it is no longer necessary to perform a colostomy.

On the rare occasions when a colostomy is considered, it should be performed about 2 weeks before planned closure, but may exceptionally be done at the time of the repair if unexpected difficulties occur (see Chapter 13).

Sometimes, a patient is seen very soon after her birth trauma, and examination reveals a large sloughing VVF and rectal defect. These patients are usually unable to walk because of nerve damage. It is controversial whether a colostomy is advisable in this situation. It has been traditional to perform one in the hope that this will make it easier to care for the patient. However, as colostomy bags are usually not available, it will not make any difference. When the time comes to perform the repair, the rectal fistula may be much smaller – and thus it turns out that a colostomy would not have been necessary. Many colostomies performed in these circumstances may never be closed.

We now hardly ever perform colostomies, although we still see some that were done elsewhere before the patient came to us.

Performing a colostomy

If a colostomy is necessary, I prefer that it be made with the pelvic colon. It should be performed through a lower midline laparotomy, bringing the proximal pelvic colon out through a small defect to the left of the umbilicus, just through the lateral rectus sheath. This minimizes the risk of colostomy prolapse. In the cases that we have seen performed by other surgeons in Africa, the main reasons for prolapse are that the transverse colon has been used or that the stoma has been brought out through too large a hole lateral to the rectus muscle.

To minimize the risk of prolapse, we recommend the following steps:

1. Use the pelvic colon.
2. Make a separate lower midline incision.
3. Choose the proximal pelvic colon where it is not too mobile.
4. Bring a loop out through a small defect that comes through the rectus muscle. The defect in the skin and rectus sheath (the rectus fibres are split) should be just enough to admit two thumbs comfortably.
5. The bowel loop should be secured in position over a firm plastic rod, and the bowel should be opened transversely and immediately sutured to skin. The rod is removed after 10 days.

A massive prolapsed colostomy is a disaster (Figure 7.2). If the RVF cannot be closed, the only solution is to close the transverse colostomy and perform a definitive end-pelvic colostomy.

Strategy for repair of a double fistula

Whenever possible, the RVF and the VVF should be repaired at the same visit to the operating theatre. It does not matter which is repaired first. Probably, most surgeons start with the bladder repair, but there is no reason why the RVF should not be done

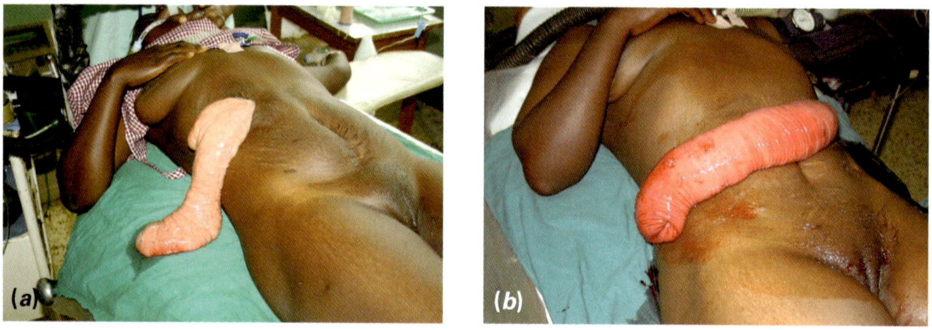

Figure 7.2 (*a, b*) Two cases of massive colostomy prolapse.

first. If this proves demanding, the bladder repair can be deferred. Most double fistulae will have a degree of vaginal stenosis, so wide relaxing incisions and episiotomies are needed. There may be difficulty in covering either of the defects, so the final decision about closure of the vagina may be left until both have been repaired.

Preoperative preparation

It is desirable that both the rectum and left colon be empty. My practice is to allow fluids only on the day before operation and to give an enema as well. An oral purgative such as sodium picosulphate (Picolax) or mannitol is very helpful. Before the anaesthetic is administered, a check should be made that the rectum is empty – if it is not then the operation should be deferred.

Technique

As for VVF repair, the first essential is very good exposure (Figure 7.3).

The repair of a simple low RVF is illustrated in Figure 7.4. This was caused by trauma in an under-age marriage.

At the Addis Ababa Fistula Hospital, where the surgeons have the greatest experience of RVF, the operative field is kept clear by swabbing by an assistant, but I find that suction is helpful, as blood accumulates in the operative field. It also helps to reduce the Trendelenberg tilt for the high fistulae.

When adequate exposure has been achieved, an incision is made around the fistula. For a small mobile fistula, it is useful to pass a Foley catheter through the defect, blow up the balloon and pull on it to bring the fistula margins into view. However, many RVFs are surrounded by varying degrees of scarring, and this approach does not work. It may be helpful to add T extensions (Figure 7.5) to the lateral margins so that a large inferior and superior flap of vaginal skin can be developed.

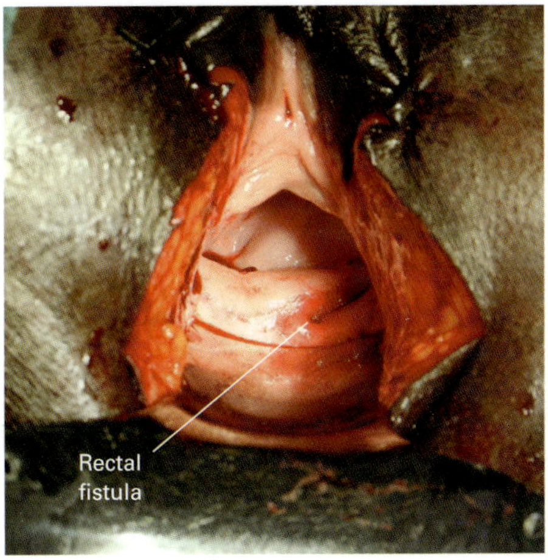

Figure 7.3 A bilateral episiotomy has been used to expose this RVF in the mid-vagina.

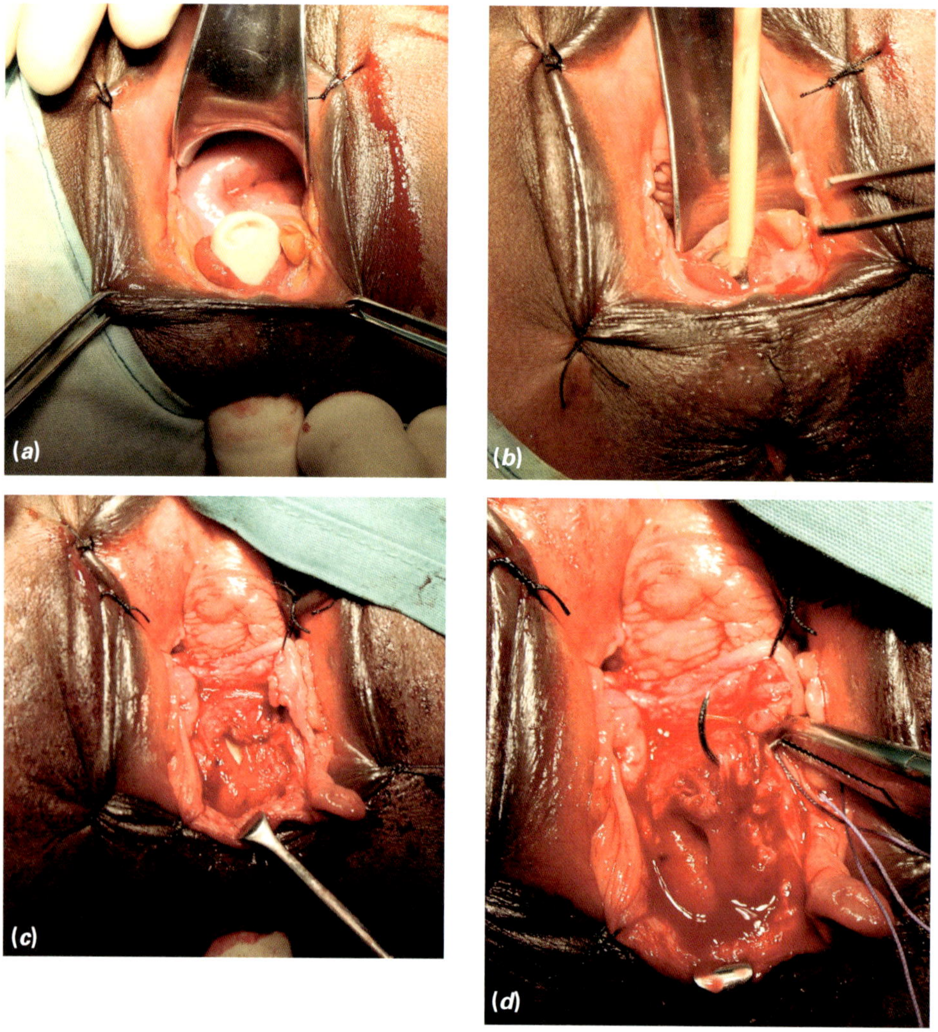

Figure 7.4 (*a*) A simple low recto-vaginal fistula. (*b*) A Foley catheter is used to expose the mobile fistula. (*c*) The vagina is separated from the rectum. (*d*) Full-thickness bites of rectal wall are taken, avoiding the rectal mucosa.

Continued

The lateral margins are the most difficult to mobilize, as they are frequently bound by scar. Generous vaginotomies may lead one into the pararectal space just below the fistula. Bold cutting with strong scissors is required to free up scar, and it helps to insert a finger frequently into the lumen of the rectum through the anus to guide the dissection.

As the posterior vaginal wall is shortened, the pouch of Douglas is often opened during the superior dissection. This is an advantage, as the rectum becomes more mobile and assessable. Significant bleeding during a rectal dissection indicates that one has strayed into the rectal wall.

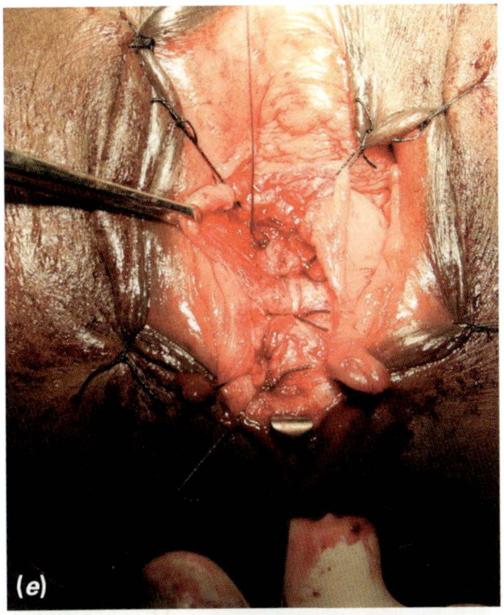

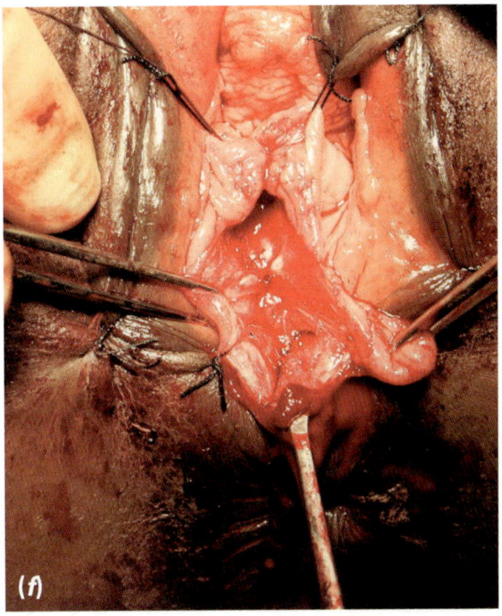

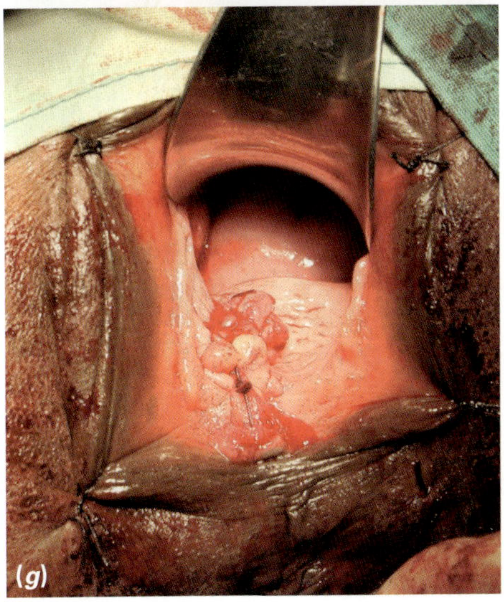

Figure 7.4 (*e*) The first layer is completed. (*f*) The second layer is completed. (*g*) The vaginal defect is closed.

It is usually appropriate to close the rectal defect transversely, and it is probably best to aim for two layers. Placing sutures accurately in a difficult RVF is not easy, so the second layer will give extra security (5/8-circle needles are most helpful). If a colostomy is present then a good single layer is sufficient.

After the repair has been completed, it is essential to check that the lumen is adequate by palpation per rectum. As the rectum is a capacious organ, a degree of narrowing is acceptable, provided that it will admit two fingers. Exceptionally, the rectum is so stenosed on initial assessment that it requires a complete resection and end-to-end anastomosis. One surgeon at the Addis Ababa Fistula Hospital has

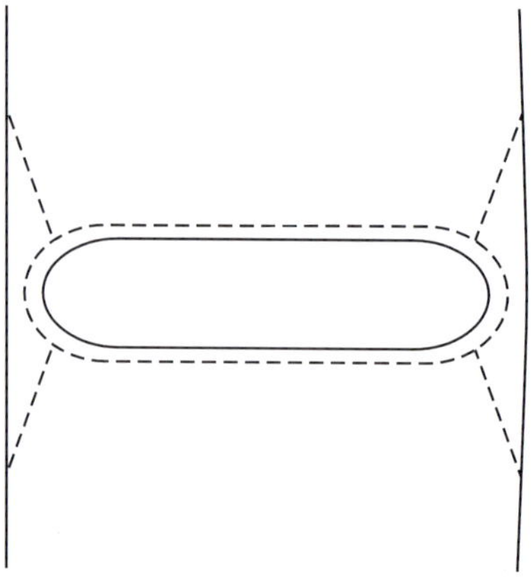

Figure 7.5 The incision around the fistula is shown by the dashed line. T extensions are made at each end.

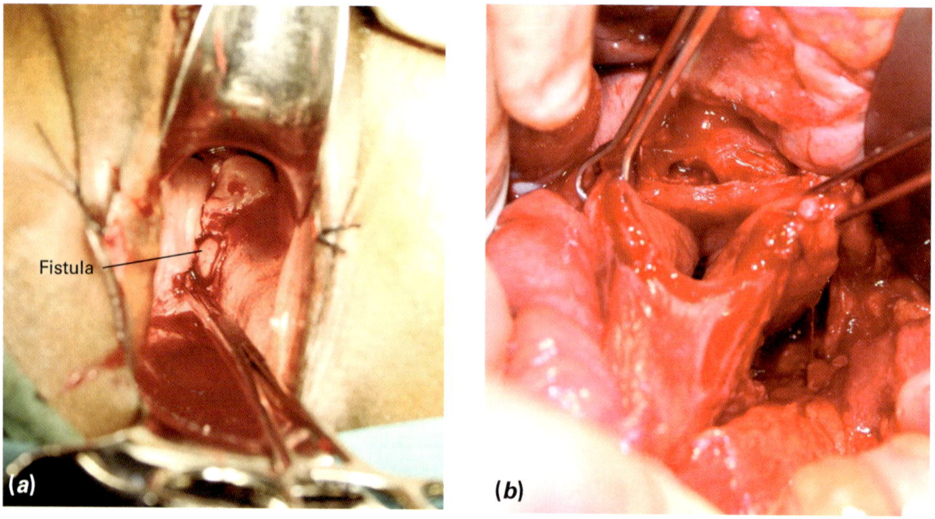

Figure 7.6 (*a*) An isolated high RVF seen vaginally. (*b*) The defect has been exposed by an abdominal approach, and is ready for suture.

developed the skill of performing this resection entirely trans-vaginally. This is very demanding, and this surgeon's particular skill has been developed only through much experience following from referrals of most of the serious RVF cases.

Some surgeons would consider a purely abdominal approach. For an experienced colorectal surgeon working in ideal conditions, a resection and end-to-end anastomosis is not difficult. However, in the average African operating theatre, this is quite another matter. It is important to appreciate that the usual bloodless fascial plane that is used to dissect the rectum and mesorectum out of the pelvis will be obliterated by scar at the site of the fistula. There is a real risk of opening the rectum where it is densely adherent to the sacrum, or of entering the presacral veins during this dissection. (The emergency management of presacral bleeding is to use a sterile drawing pin. It is pushed through the bleeder into the sacrum – it will do no harm. Failing this, one has to pack and come out.)

Given the conditions that exist in many African hospitals, an abdominal approach is not recommended as the first line. The exception was at the Addis Ababa Fistula Hospital, where I have seen two exceptional case of isolated very high fistulae adherent to the sacral promontory. These were out of reach vaginally, but were quite easily closed by an abdominal approach, which also allowed simultaneous closure of the pre-existing colostomies (Figure 7.6).

There are occasions where I have found a combined approach very helpful. In spite of persistent mobilization from below, I have not felt able to close a defect high in the rectum securely. After opening the abdomen, it was quite easy to complete the repair from above, as most of the mobilization had already been done (Figure 7.7).

Results of rectal repairs

It is most surgeons' experience that the results of repair are good, although we do not know how many cases are turned down because of severe injury. Exceptionally, I see a patient with an RVF and bladder injuries so bad that I consider them inoperable. Given ideal operating conditions, I might have been able to operate on some of these patients.

I classify one-third of RVFs as high, and prefer to repair these first, sometimes deferring the VVF repair to a later date. Of these high cases, I close half vaginally and the other half by a combined approach. In the Addis Ababa Fistula Hospital, I have closed five specially selected cases entirely from the abdomen.

In cases with a low- to mid-level RVF, I almost always close the bladder defect at the same visit to the operating theatre. Of my 47 rectal repairs, only 2 required a second repair, and 1 was so bad that she was left with a permanent colostomy.

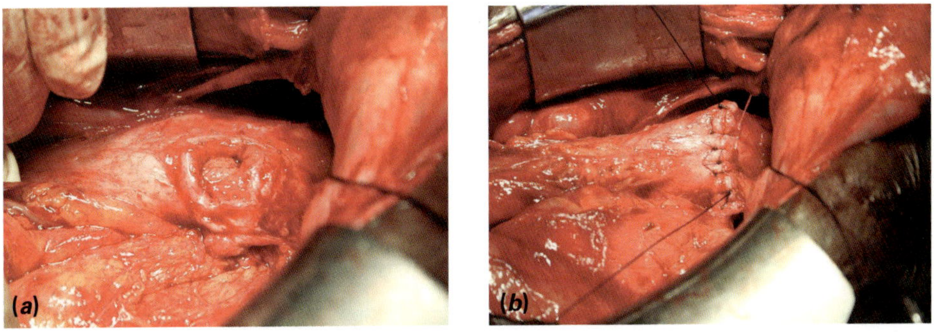

Figure 7.7 (a) A high RVF started from below and completed from above. The fistula margins are trimmed and ready for suture. (*b*) The defect has been closed with a single layer of inverting sutures.

The success rate for the concomitant bladder repair was much worse. Less than 50% were discharged dry. These poor results reflect the severe injury in the region of the bladder neck that so often accompanies an RVF. It is rare to find a juxta-cervical fistula in association with an RVF.

Finally, it must be emphasized that surgery for RVF is demanding, and should not be undertaken lightly by inexperienced surgeons. Only the low fistulae are relatively easy.

References

1. Kelly J, Kwast BE. Epidemiological study of vesico-vaginal fistula in Ethiopia. *Int Urogynaecol J* 1993; **4**: 278–81.
2. Muleta M, Williams G. Post coital injuries treated at the Addis Ababa Fistula hospital 1991–1997. *Lancet* 1999; **354**: 2051–2.
3. Goh J, Krause H. *Female Genital Tract Fistula*. Brisbane: University of Queensland Press, 2004.

8 Repair of Anal Sphincter Injuries

Immediate repair

Anal sphincter tears seen within 24 hours of delivery should be repaired at once. This is not a minor operation. The patient's future continence depends on the skill of the repair.

It is important when carrying out the repair to realize that torn anal sphincters retract to the 3 and 9 o'clock position.

The repair must be carried out in an operating theatre with good lighting, instruments and assistance. Repair under local anaesthesia is possible, but it is be better to have the patient under a spinal or general anaesthetic. The patient should come to theatre with an empty rectum.

The ano-rectal mucosa are closed first; then the torn ends of the external sphincter are identified (the internal sphincter cannot be identified as a separate layer). These ends are sutured accurately, taking quite big bites using a slowly absorbable suture (Vicryl or Dexon). Three to four sutures are needed. The vagina and perineal skin are then closed, using good mattress sutures to build up the perineal body.

Secondary repair

If the repair cannot be performed immediately, it is best to wait for several weeks. Sometimes, patients with an old complete tear say that they have no symptoms, so it is important to be sure that a patient really does have troublesome faecal leakage before recommending repair. In the best hands, only 80% of repairs restore complete continence.

Again, it is important to realize that the torn ends of the sphincter have retracted round half the anal circumference, and simply freshening the margins of the tear and suturing them is unlikely to give a good result. The procedure is illustrated in Figure 8.1.

The patient is usually kept on fluids only for the first two postoperative days. A mild laxative can be given on the third day.

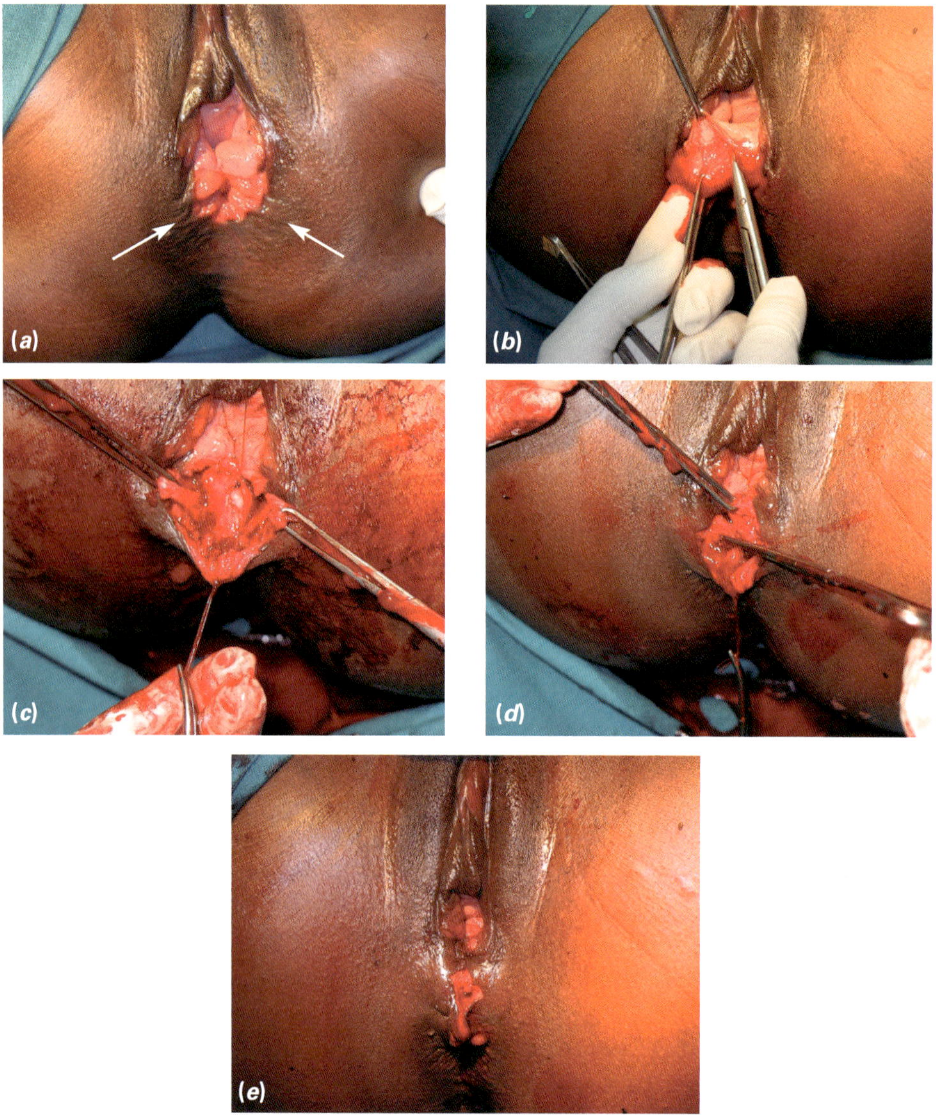

Figure 8.1 (*a*) A late complete anal sphincter tear. The arrows indicate the position of the retracted sphincter ends. (*b*) The vaginal mucosa is separated from the rectal mucosa well above the tear. Then the ends of the sphincter are identified postero-laterally. A block of tissue that contains the sphincter end should be mobilized. If only muscle is mobilized, it will easily tear. (*c*) The ano-rectal mucosa has been repaired, and blocks of tissue containing the external sphincter are held in forceps. (*d*) The aim is to repair the sphincters by overlapping the two blocks of tissue. The mobilized tissue should contain some scar tissue around the sphincter. Pure sphincter muscle would not hold sutures well. (*e*) The completed repair. The initial transverse incision has been converted to a vertical one. There is tension in the middle of the suture line, so the wound has been left open here. Should infection or bleeding occur, the repair would not be compromised.

9 Management of Post-repair Incontinence

Introduction

It is one thing to be able to close a vesico-vaginal fistula, but it is another matter to make patients continent. We can close over 90% of cases, but another 20% at least will have some incontinence, and in about half it is so bad that the patient is still totally wet. This 'incontinence gap' is a source of great frustration to fistula surgeons. Its cause is not hard to see.

The mid-urethra may be more important than the urethro-vesical junction in maintaining continence. In our series, 35% of patients have a fistula less than 2.5 cm from the external urethral orifice (i.e. one involving the mid-urethra) and 60% have a fistula within 4 cm of the orifice (i.e. involving the urethro-vesical junction). In addition to being shortened, the urethra may be denervated, fibrosed and functionless.

Bladder function may be disturbed in several ways. The bladder size can range from normal to severely reduced. Its compliance can vary, ranging from being atonic with chronic retention and overflow to unstable with frequent abnormal pressure waves (detrusor instability, leading to urge incontinence). If these variables could be identified by urodynamic testing they could help us with management. Our studies in fistula patients are in their infancy.

Andrew Browning has developed a special interest in the management of stress, and this chapter will focus on his preferred operative procedure and management. This is a combination of urethral and bladder neck plication and the use of a fibro-muscular sling. Other surgeons have different approaches, and, although we have limited experience of these, they will be briefly discussed later in the chapter.

The management of post-repair stress incontinence falls under four headings:

- immediate assessment
- conservative measures
- surgical management
- management with a urethral plug.

Immediate assessment

Frequency and poor control are common just after catheter removal, but often improve rapidly. If the patient is still wet after 48 hours, and assuming that a dye test has excluded a breakdown, she needs to be categorized into one of four degrees of severity:

- *Wet with exertion (coughing or effort).* This often improves over time with pelvic floor exercises.
- *Wet on walking, dry on sitting and lying, but can void well.* Again, this can often improve with time and pelvic floor exercises.
- *Wet on walking, sitting and lying, but still able to void to some extent.* This does not often improve with time, and the patient will either need assistance with a urethral plug or a secondary stress operation, usually after 6 months of trial of pelvic floor exercises.
- *Wet all the time, not voiding.* This rarely improves with time. It is often due to a very small bladder and/or a functionless urethra. A urethral plug may be of benefit if the urethra is not too lax. Over time, intermittent occlusion of the urethra may help to expand the bladder, and a secondary stress procedure can then help. Patients who do well with the plug usually do well with a secondary stress operation.

Conservative management – pelvic floor exercises

In developed countries, there is objective evidence that pelvic floor exercises are of value in the management of stress incontinence. But the benefit has only been shown in motivated patients who have had proper instruction from a professional.

Great importance has been placed in the instruction of fistula patients in pelvic floor exercises. Unfortunately, the women with the worst stress incontinence are those who have ischaemic damage to the pelvic floor muscles. One has only to put two fingers in the vagina, and feel the fibrosis in the vagina and levator muscles and ask the patient to squeeze, to realize how little contraction there is.

Other patients with stress but with less damage will benefit from instruction – but only if this is done properly (Figure 9.1). It is essential to put two fingers in the vagina to help the patient to understand what to do and to check on progress. Simple verbal instruction is doomed to failure. The patient should also be taught to examine herself for feedback.

The routine taught at the Addis Ababa Fistula Hospital is for the patient to tighten her pelvic floor as strongly as possible for 5–10 seconds. She should continue to breathe normally. The squeeze is then repeated 10–20 times, with gaps of 10 seconds between. The patient should repeat this routine three times a day.

A happy event is that we sometimes see patients going home with moderate stress, but returning later to tell us that the incontinence has cleared up spontaneously after a few weeks.

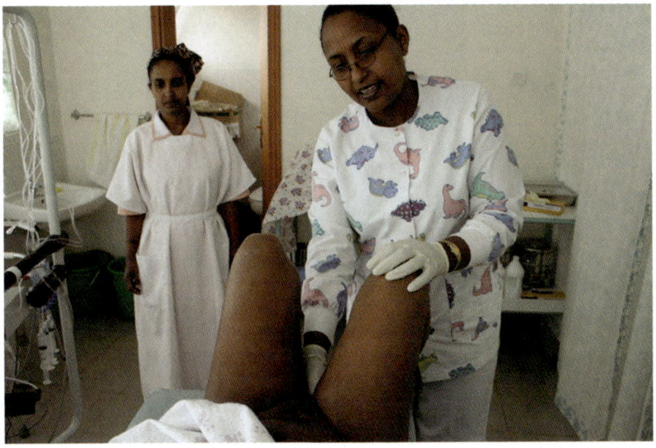

Figure 9.1 Teaching pelvic floor exercises at the Addis Ababa Fistula Hospital.

Surgical management

At least 6 months should pass to allow time for spontaneous improvement. A secondary stress incontinence procedure can then be considered. First, the diagnosis must be confirmed and a dye test performed again. *It is very easy to overlook a tiny residual fistula.* The test should be done in theatre at the start of any proposed stress operation. If it is negative, incontinence can be demonstrated by removing the catheter with the dye still inside it: often, the dye just gushes out – if it does not, the patient should be asked to cough, whereupon incontinence is usually readily appreciated.

Until recently a simple cystometry was performed to aid selection. The bladder was filled with water through an open bladder syringe held vertically while compressing the urethra. If the bladder pressure was estimated to be more than 20 cmH_2O with only 100 cm^3 in the bladder, operation was not recommended. This excluded about one-third of patients. Now, all patients are given a chance with the plication and sling, and the success rate (around two-thirds) has decreased only slightly.

Urethral plication with a fibro-muscular sling

The aim of the surgery is to lengthen and narrow the urethra and then provide support with a fibro-muscular sling (the sling is described and illustrated in Chapter 6).

Position the patient as for a fistula repair, and use an episiotomy if necessary. First, measure the length of the urethra as follows: insert a Foley catheter; inflate the balloon; pull the catheter until the balloon abuts the bladder neck; pinch the catheter at the level of the external urethral meatus; deflate the balloon; remove the Foley while still pinching it; re-inflate the balloon. The urethral length is from where the Foley is pinched to the balloon (Figure 9.2a). In Ethiopia, the average length before operation is 1.4 cm, which is less than half the normal length. Almost all patients will have a shortened urethra.

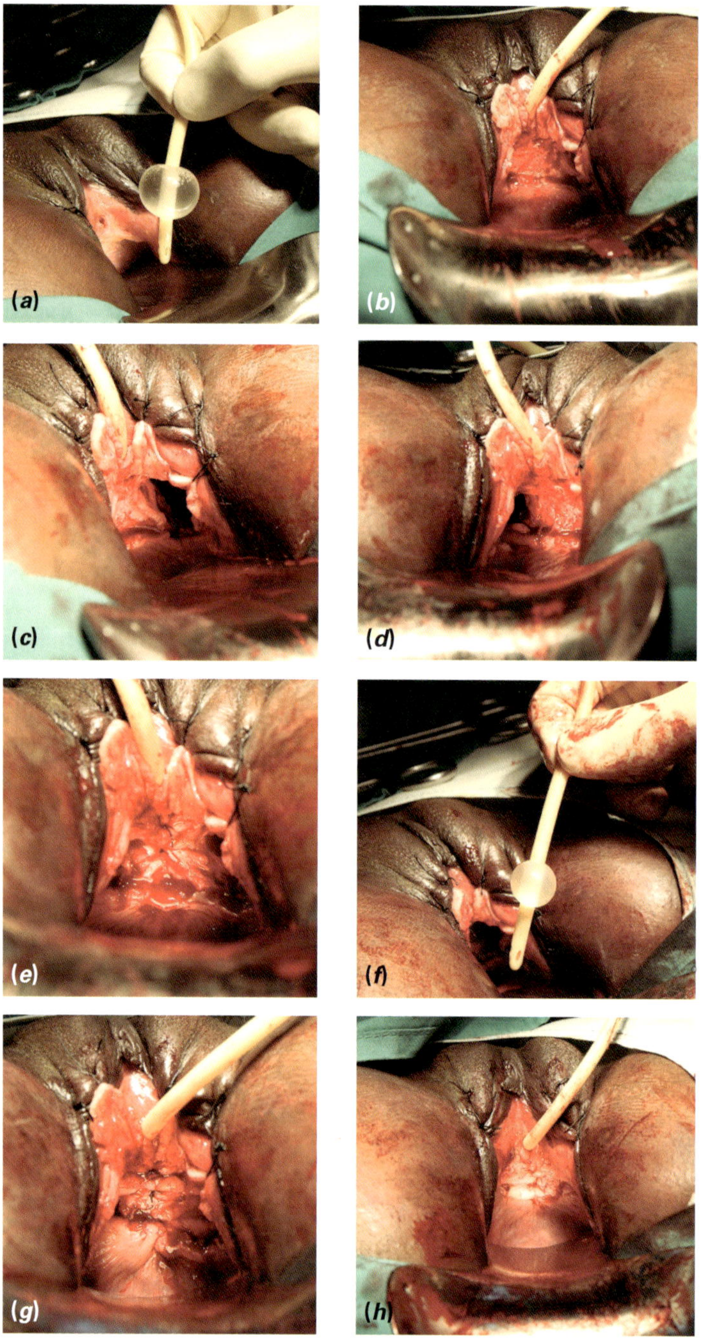

Figure 9.2 Urethral plication with a fibro-muscular sling. (*a*) The urethral length is 1.5 cm. (*b*) The vaginal flaps are elevated. (*c*) The right para-vesical space is opened. (*d*) The left para-vesical space is opened. (*e*) Plication has been completed. (*f*) The urethral length is now 3 cm. (*g*) The fibro-muscular sling is made over the plicated urethra. (*h*) The vaginal incision is closed.

Next, reflect the vagina mucosa. Make a vertical incision through the vagina along the urethra, with a metal catheter in situ, beginning just proximal to the external urethral meatus. This incision should be the length that you would like the urethra to be: about 3–4 cm, Make the incision into an inverted 'T' incision, with the arms of the 'T' extending onto the lateral vaginal walls. Reflect these flaps either side, and suture them out of the way to the labia majora (Figure 9.2b). Dissect a little under the horizontal incision to mobilize the distal bladder. With scissors, dissect the urethra and bladder off from the lateral attachments, opening the para-vesical space on either side (Figure 9.2c, d).

Great care should be taken, as it is easy to open the bladder here and create another fistula. If this happens, it is usually because the first operation was for a circumferential fistula that was not repaired in a circumferential manner. Re-repair is extremely difficult, but must be attempted.

The next step is to plicate the urethra and distal bladder with three or four interrupted sutures in the midline. These aim to pick up the pubo-cervical fascia, or at least its remnants, to narrow the urethra and pull the walls of the distal bladder together. This has the effect of producing a lumen inside that will have its diameter narrowed to resemble that of the urethra (Figure 9.2e).

Measure the length of the urethra again to see if it has lengthened. The average length of the urethra had doubled to 3 cm in the Ethiopia series of 72 consecutive cases (Figure 9.2f).

Perform a dye test to ensure that the bladder has not been opened accidentally.

Make a sling by grasping the fibro-muscular tissue on each side, developing a block of tissue to be sutured together in the midline (Figure 9.2g). Of course, a sling may have been made at the primary operation, but additional tissue can usually be found to make another one. Note that there may be brisk bleeding as the pedicle is elevated. This can be a source of postoperative bleeding if it is not carefully attended to.

The vagina is now repaired (Figure 9.2h). Take a deep bite though the lateral vaginal incision to include the bed of the pedicle. This reduces any dead space and bleeding.

The Foley catheter is left on free drainage for 3 days, and the patient is encouraged to drink as usual. After removal of the catheter, the patient is encouraged to void every 2 hours. After 2 days, the residual urine after voiding should be measured. It should be less than 100 cm^3. If it is not, the patient is deemed to have urinary retention, which needs treatment – see below. The patient is also shown how to perform pelvic floor exercises. The patient is assessed, and any remaining stress is quantified into the scale referred to previously so see if there has been any improvement from before the operation.

Complications

Complications of this procedure include:

- accidental re-opening of the fistula in about 5% of cases
- ligation of ureters if the sutures have been placed too deep (this has not been recognized in our experience)
- retention of urine in 15% of cases.

Management of retention

A few patients cannot pass urine at all and must have the catheter re-inserted; others have a degree of retention that, if undetected, could lead to overflow incontinence, urinary tract infection and even stone formation.

All patients should have their residual urine measured before being allowed home. If it is more than 100 cm^3, proceed as follows:

- Replace the catheter, and repeat the measurement in 48 hours.
- If the residual urine is still more than 100 cm^3, teach the patient double voiding. In this, the patient voids as normal, perhaps with supra-pubic pressure – pushing on this area with her hand. She then stands up and walks around for a few moments while the bladder 'readjusts' to having a smaller volume of urine in it, and then she tries to void again.
- If this does not fix the problem after another 48 hours, teach her clean intermittent self-catheterization. She should try to void as much as she can and then pass a short stiff catheter into her bladder to drain the remaining urine. She washes the catheter and keeps it clean to use the next time. Most patients will improve in time, although there may be a small group in whom the bladder never regains the capacity to empty, so self-catheterization may be for life. In this case, the patient should be provided with a metal catheter.

We have heard from one surgeon that the incidence of retention will be reduced it the catheter is left in for 10 days post operation rather than 3 days as we practise. This requires further investigation.

Results

These have been promising in the short term.[1] Two-thirds of patients went home dry. This includes a few who needed to be taught self-catheterization for retention. Of the remaining one-third, half were improved (from being wet all the time to wet only with coughing or wet on walking), and some of the others gained benefit from using a urethral plug.

My experience with only 24 operations of plication and sling is not quite as good as that of Andrew Browning. In a few patients, I cannot find any tissue for a sling, so just do a plication. Sometimes, this is barely possible because of fibrosis. It is difficult for a visiting surgeon to know his results compared with a resident one. Approximately half of my patients are reported as dry after catheter removal, and I have not been aware of retention as a problem – but this could well have been overlooked. I have only once re-opened a fistula. It is possible that I have not been radical enough in performing the plication and sling. I still use this as my first choice for severe stress, as the operation is relatively easy to do and does not preclude other procedures such as fascial slings later.

The procedure clearly shows promise, but time will tell if others can reproduce Andrew Browning's very encouraging results.

Other stress procedures

Ideally, urodynamic assessment should both help us to understand the cause and help in selection of surgery. It was available at the Addis Ababa Fistula Hospital to Carey and colleagues when they first introduced the rectus facial sling there.[2]

A random group of incontinent patients were assessed urodynamically. Only 41% were found to have genuine stress incontinence with a compliant bladder. A similar percentage were found to have detrusor instability as well, which was thought to be a contraindication to surgery; the remainder had either a very small bladder or retention with overflow. Only the first group had the operation. Of these, 78% were dry on discharge, although some relapses were seen later.

Good urodynamic facilities continue to be used at the Addis Ababa Fistula Hospital to select patients for the rectus fascial sling, which is the preferred operative method there. At present, only patients with a bladder capacity of 200 cm^3 or more are accepted. About 70% of patients with serious stress fulfil these criteria. Small capacity of the bladder rather than bladder wall instability appears the main contraindication in the other 30%; they are managed with urethral plugs where possible. In the hands of one surgeon who specializes in this procedure, at least 40% of these selected cases appear cured and another 40% considerably improved. Publication of the results of these urodynamic studies and the surgical outcomes is anxiously awaited.

For the vast majority of surgeons working without urodynamic facilities, some simple observations can be made that may help in selection. We are indebted to David Lyth working at the Aberdeen Clinic and Fistula Centre in Freetown, Sierra Leone, for the following suggestions. First, patients can be asked to wear pads for 24 hours to get an idea of the amount of wetness, and any urine voided in that time should be measured. Residual urine should be measured in the un-anaesthetized patient, and the bladder capacity is measured by gradually filling the bladder though an open syringe held 20 cm above the level of the bladder. Provided that there was no pre-existing retention, a good bladder capacity (250 cm^3) is a favourable sign. The catheter is removed, leaving the fluid inside. If it then squirts out, this suggests an unstable bladder – a predictor of a poorer operative outcome. On the other hand, those patients in whom there is leakage only on coughing should do better. The best prognostic sign for a successful rectus sling operation is a good result using a urethral plug.

We have little personal experience of this operation. The principle is illustrated in Figure 9.3. A strip of rectus fascia is taken via a supra-pubic incision and passed under the urethra. The dissection is started under the mid-urethra, passing laterally on each side into the retro-pubic space. Forceps are passed behind the pubis, pressing hard against bone to minimize the risk of opening the bladder, until the rectus sheath is reached. Strong sutures attached to each end of the fascial strip are used to manoeuvre the sling through this tunnel and under the urethra. It is then sutured to the rectus sheath just above the pubis. There is general agreement that the sling should be pulled up more tightly than one would for patients in developed countries. A guide is that it should be tight enough for a 14 Fr catheter to encounter significant resistance. Over-tightening may predispose to retention, but patients may prefer to self-catheterize than be wet.

There are many ways of performing the operation that are described in standard operative textbooks of urology or gynaecology, but it should be appreciated that in patients in developed countries the urethra is substantially intact, whereas in fistula patients requiring surgery it is usually short, surrounded by fibrosis and functionless. Methods applicable to fistula patients are described by Judith Goh and Hannah Krause in their book[3] and by Michael Breen in his lecture notes.[4]

Kees Waaldijk, who has vast experience of fistula surgery in Northern Nigeria, has evolved his own operation for stress incontinence, which has been used in over 500 cases. This involves a radical plication of urethra and bladder base – even more so than in Andrew Browning's operation. A form of colpo-suspension is then performed in which the bladder base is hitched up, using the remaining pubo-cervical fascia, to the arcus tendinus region on the pelvic side wall. All this is done from below through the widely opened para-vesical space, using an aneurysm needle

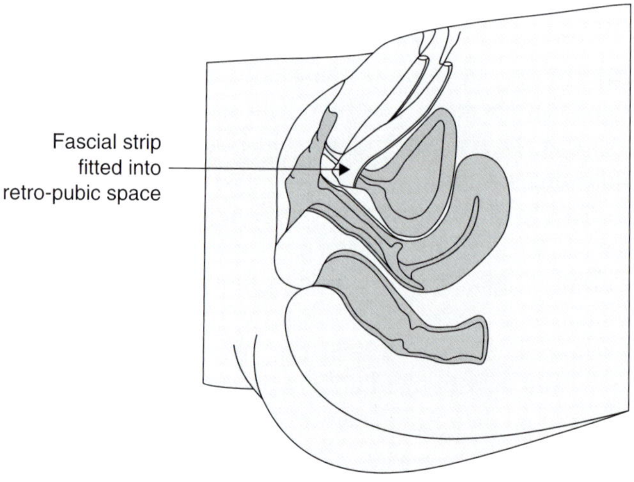

Figure 9.3 Rectus fascial sling in position.

for access. This has worked well for Waaldijk, with up to 60% of selected patients being completely dry. However, this method has not been widely used by others.

Finally, it should be mentioned that some enthusiastic visiting surgeons have performed tension-free tape operations on selected patients. The trans-obturator method has been favoured because such good results are reported in non-fistula patients. However, our fistula patients are young, usually with scarred, rigid, shortened urethras – quite different from patients in developed countries. It is not surprising that several unsatisfactory results have occurred, with a serious risk of later erosion of the tape. We see no place for its use on a casual basis.

Only a few surgeons are regularly operating for stress incontinence. Clearly, the problem of post-repair incontinence is a major one, and there is an urgent need for full-time fistula surgeons to report selection criteria and results – both good and bad. Whatever procedure is adopted, it is probably only the full-time fistula surgeons who take an interest in this problem who will achieve good results. At present, in the best hands, only 50% of patients who are wet post-repair can be made dry, and we know nothing of long-term results. Improvements may come when we learn how to select patients better by simple observation and measurements and can define the best surgical procedures.

Urethral plug

The urethral plug is a small, simple device that, as the name suggests, merely plugs the urethra to stop urine draining out (Figure 9.4). It can be used for any patient who is still severely bothered by her incontinence.

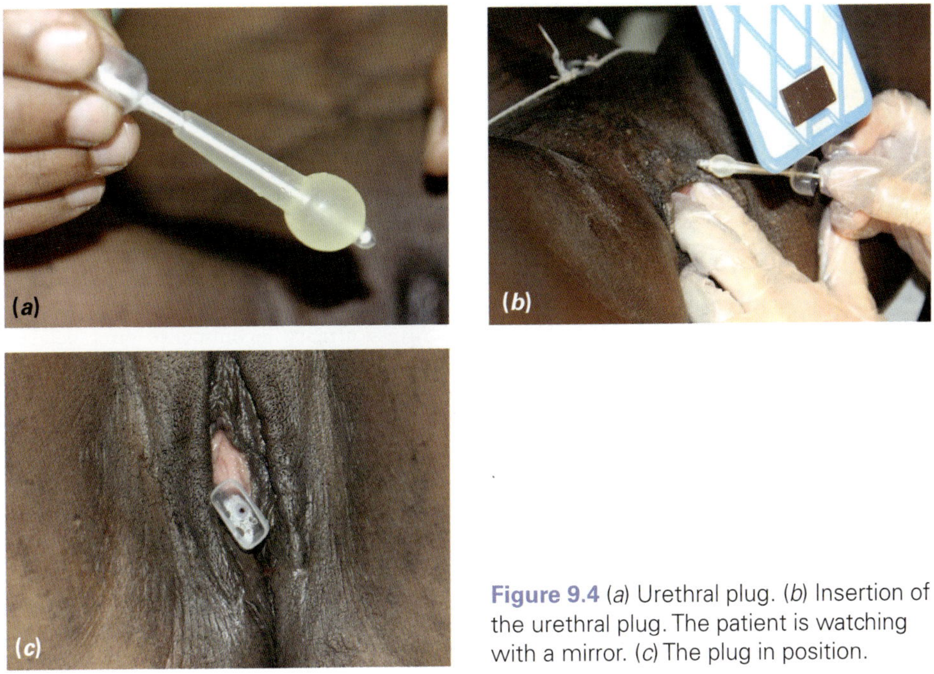

Figure 9.4 (*a*) Urethral plug. (*b*) Insertion of the urethral plug. The patient is watching with a mirror. (*c*) The plug in position.

There are a few patients in whom plugs will not work. These are usually patients with very small bladders or very wide urethras.

The plug is inserted into the urethra with the aid of an introducer. The patient should be able to do this quite easily herself after a few lessons. She may be helped by using a small hand-held mirror. The introducer is removed after insertion and kept in a safe place. When she feels urine in the bladder or urine starts to leak around the plug, often signalling a full bladder, the introducer is put back inside the plug to allow its withdrawal.

With increasing experience of plugs, Andrew Browning has seen some patients in whom there has been a demonstrable increase in bladder size over time and who have stopped using the plug because they are continent.

Some risks are involved with use of urethral plugs, namely infection and trauma to the urethra causing bleeding and pain. To minimize these, the patient is told to use the plug for only 12 hours a day – either all night or all day, but not both.

There have also been reports of plugs being lost in the bladder. Where an operating cystoscope was not available, the plug had to removed by open cystotomy.

The plug is meant to be a single-use device, but, owing to its cost, this is clearly not possible in the developing world. The patient is taught to clean it with soap once a day and to wash it after each application, along with increasing the amount of fluid that she drinks. This reduces the chance of infection, and one plug can last up to about a month with this regime. The patient can return for follow-up and assessment if she needs more plugs.

Urethral plugs have a role to play in the management of intractable incontinence, but can be safely used only in the setting of a permanent fistula unit. Plugs are used at the Addis Ababa Fistula Hospital and its satellite centres and the Aberdeen Clinic and Fistula Centre in Freetown. Further studies from these centres on longer-term use of plugs are awaited with interest.

References

1. Browning A. A new technique for the surgical management of urinary incontinence after obstetric fistula repair. *Br J Obstet Gynaecol* 2006; **113**: 475–8.
2. Carey MP, Goh J, Fynes MM, Murray CJ. Stress urinary incontinence after delayed primary closure of genitourinary fistulae: a technique for surgical management. *Am J Obstet Gynecol* 2002; **186**: 948–53.
3. Goh J, Krause H. *Female Genital Tract Fistula*. Brisbane: University of Queensland Press, 2004.
4. Breen M. *Teaching Notes for Obstetric Fistula Repair*. CD, available from Michael Breen, Monze Hospital, PO Box 660029, Monze, Zambia (mbreen@zamnet.zm).

10 Management of the Inoperable Case

Inevitably, there are cases where the injuries are so extreme that no surgeon, however skilful, can make the patient continent. The most common of these situations is virtually complete loss of bladder tissue (Figure 10.1). Another is stenosis of the vagina so severe as to preclude any assessment or attempt at cure. A rare case is a patient so obese that it is impossible to see or access the fistula. Occasionally, a patient presents with severe generalized illness (e.g. a low immune state) that makes repair futile.

In the majority of cases, inoperability is caused by multiple factors, the most important being failed previous repair in combination with a damaged urethra, a small bladder and severe fibrosis. Other patients have total incontinence following a failed operation for stress.

What can be offered to these patients? If urethral plugs are available, they must be tried if the problem is stress, but, failing that, there are only two options: do nothing or perform some form of urinary diversion.

Before considering any of the possible procedures, there are some serious questions to be considered. Any form of diversion is a major procedure, with significant immediate and long-term morbidity. It is also irreversible. There may be enormous pressure on a fistula surgeon to 'do something for the poor woman' – not only from the patient herself, but also from the other members of the team who hate having to turn away a patient and say that nothing more can be done. There may be

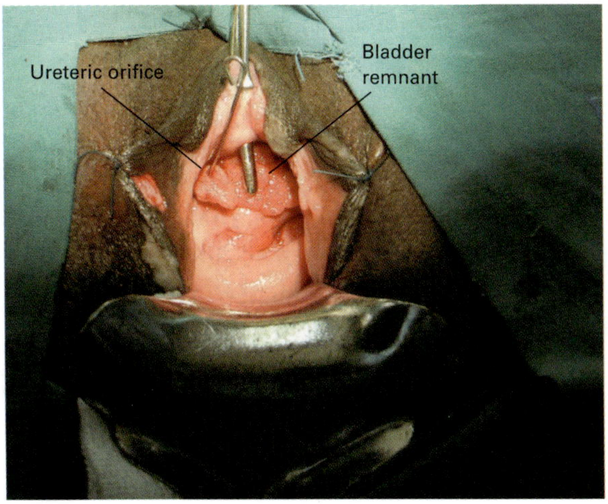

Figure 10.1 A tiny remnant of bladder, with a probe in the right ureteric orifice.

well-intentioned visiting surgeons who are skilled in pelvic surgery in their home setting and who believe that they can contribute their technical skill to perform complex operations. It must be said here that, for all their good intentions, they may do more harm than good.[1]

Before a diversion is performed, many criteria have to be satisfied:

- Is the case truly inoperable? Only a skilled fistula surgeon working regularly in Africa can make that judgement. Of course, there are so few of these that it may be impossible for the patient to be so assessed.
- Do the patient and her family understand what is proposed, and have the possible benefits and risks been understood? Often, the surgeon and patient are separated by culture, skin colour and language, and their social conditions, beliefs, customs and knowledge of the functioning of the human body may be incomprehensible to each other.
- If these hurdles are overcome and the patient consents, are the conditions in the theatre and for aftercare sufficient to conduct major surgery safely? Who will care for the few patients who will inevitably develop some life-threatening complications if a surgeon is not available? Who will be responsible for long-term follow-up?

We believe that there are circumstances where diversion procedures are appropriate, but they should be performed only by surgeons who are working long term in a developing country and who can be responsible for aftercare and follow-up. We believe that they have an obligation to obtain follow-up and report their results honestly, as we know so little about the quality of life after diversion procedures. It is very tempting for surgeons to report only their successes – but those working with fistula patients need to know about the failures as well.

The possibilities for diversion are briefly discussed here.

The ileal conduit

This involves wearing a urostomy bag for life. This may be the procedure of choice in the developed world, where the diversion can be performed with low morbidity and where urostomy bags are freely available. In the developing world, this is really out of the question. The exception is in the Addis Ababa Fistula Hospital, which has had the services of a skilled visiting urologist for many years. Many ileal conduits have been constructed, with a very low morbidity. The patients are completely dry, but because bags can be provided only from the hospital, these patients cannot return to their homes in remote areas. This problem has been partly overcome by providing a separate village not far from the hospital where they can live. Whether they are entirely happy with this situation is an open question. Now that a series of outreach centres have been set up, it may be possible for some patients to return home and obtain supplies of bags locally.

The continent ileal bladder

This is major 5- to 6-hour operation requiring a high degree of skill. The attractiveness is the prospect that a continent pouch of small intestine is emptied by intermittent self-catheterization. This may have an acceptable place in the developed world, but it is out of the question in Africa in view of its complexity and very significant morbidity, which would require highly skilled surgical attention.

The Mitrofanoff procedure

This involves diverting the ureters into a pouch made of isolated caecum and ascending colon. The appendix is reversed and implanted into the pouch, and is brought out in the right iliac fossa or through the umbilicus. The patient empties the pouch by self-catheterization through the appendix.

An alternative approach may be possible if the urethra is irreparable but the bladder is of good size. The bladder neck is closed and the reversed appendix is implanted into the bladder vault.

We know of patients who have had a good quality of life after these procedures, but there is a significant incidence of problems of stenosis and difficult catheterization.[2] If the patient is far away from skilled help, this is a disaster.

The Mainz pouch II

Diversion of urine into the large intestine has some merits. It is the most frequently performed diversion procedure, but there are only anecdotal reports of even short-term follow-up in Africa to guide us as to the quality of life. The operation can make the patient dry by day and often at night – but at the price of significant morbidity and risk to life expectancy.

Traditionally, the procedure involved anastomosing the ureters to the sigmoid colon. Over the last two decades, this has been modified by creating a pouch of sigmoid colon by anastomosing two loops together (the Mainz pouch II). This has the effect of creating a low-pressure reservoir, thus decreasing the frequency of passing urine per rectum and probably reducing the amount of reflux up the ureters.

Clearly, the patient is going to pass urine though the rectum for the rest of her life, and must have a near-perfect ano-rectal continence mechanism.

Four components are necessary for complete anal continence: two motor and two sensory.

On the motor side, there must be an intact internal sphincter. Its function is to keep the anal canal closed at rest. More important is a functioning external sphincter complex. It is well known in developed countries that occult injury (detected by ultrasound and electromyographic studies) occurs quite often after normal delivery, and this may be related to the length of the second stage and the size of the baby. This is usually asymptomatic, although in later life it may predispose to faecal incontinence or rectal prolapse. It is not known if this occurs in the African setting. More obvious are overt sphincter tears and, even after skilled repair, there are symptomatic defects in continence in about 20% of patients. A previous repair may preclude this diversion option.

On the sensory side, somatic sensation from the epithelium of the lower two-thirds of the anal canal provides fine discrimination of the nature of rectal contents (gas, liquid or solid), while stretch receptors in the levator ani complex provide information about the extent of distension in the rectum. Both components can be damaged by prolonged labour, either from a traction neuropathy of the pudendal nerve or ischaemia to the sacral plexus and fibrosis in the levator complex.

A degree of saddle anaesthesia and absent anal reflex may be found more often than expected if specifically looked for soon after a prolonged labour in fistula patients.[3] There has been one report of defects in anal continence that were detected unexpectedly during a study of postoperative urinary incontinence.[3]

This subject needs more objective study.

In practice, it is possible to assess the quality of sphincter function by assessing the resting anal tone (mostly contributed by the internal sphincter) and the squeeze pressure (contributed by the external anal sphincter) on digital rectal examination. An additional test is to fill the rectum with about 300 cm^3 of saline to make sure that the patient can hold it for some hours.

To perform a colonic diversion in a patient with a missed recto-vaginal fistula or defective continence mechanism is a disaster (Figure 10.2).

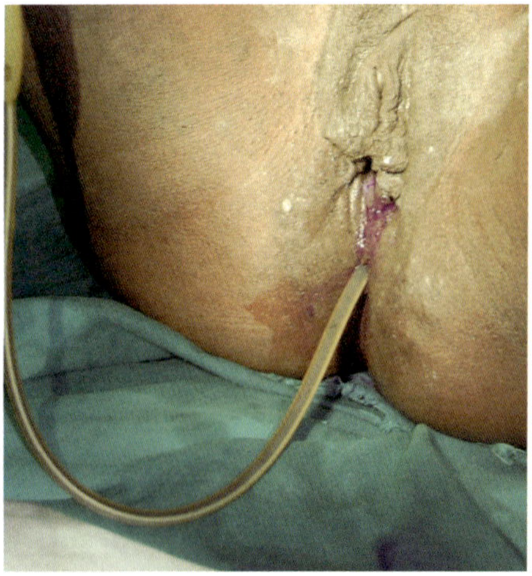

Figure 10.2 This patient had an unreparable vesico-vaginal fistula. A rectal dye test as part of a pre-pouch work-up revealed a completely unsuspected tiny recto-vaginal fistula in some posterior scar. This is an absolute contraindication to a Mainz pouch until it has been repaired.

At best, a patient having a diversion should be continent at least by day, although she may have to empty her bowel four or five times. A few patients report regular leakage at night and need to wear a pad.

The best long-term review of results from developed countries highlights a number of downsides, which may not be amenable to detection or treatment in Africa:[4]

- This is *major surgery*, with a small but significant immediate morbidity and mortality.
- *Acid–base disturbances*. Chloride and hydrogen ions destined for excretion in the urine are reabsorbed to some extent by the colonic mucosa. Provided that renal function is normal, the patient may come to no harm, although some will develop a hyperchloraemic acidosis, which may be asymptomatic for a time, but ultimately leads to thinning of bones and renal failure. Any pre-existing renal failure or repeated renal infection will speed up this deterioration. Early detection of electrolyte imbalance is important, as further deterioration can be mitigated by regular taking of sodium bicarbonate. This means measurement of acid–base balance, as changes in sodium and potassium are late indicators of the problem. Facilities for measurement of bicarbonate levels are rare in Africa. From studies in the developed world, it is thought that at least 50% of patients have evidence of mild acidosis on testing 1 year after operation, and these patients are advised to take regular alkalizing agents (sodium bicarbonate). In a few patients, there may be pre-existing renal impairment due to chronic ureteric obstruction. A raised creatinine or bilateral hydronephrosis would be a contraindication to diversion.
- *Renal infection*. Recurrent urinary infection is possible. Its incidence seems reduced by creation of a low-pressure pouch, but it is predisposed to by any stenosis at the uretero-colonic anastomosis. Thus, a good technique at surgery is critical to the subsequent outcome. Yet stenosis bad enough to require revision surgery may occur in up to 5% of cases, even in expert hands (detected by dilatation of the renal tract on ultrasound scanning).
- Diversion of urine to the colon predisposes to *development of carcinoma of the colon*. This reaches significant levels (around 20%) only if the patient should survive for more than 20 years after a conventional uretero-sigmoidostomy. It is not known if making a pouch will reduce the risk. In developed countries, a patient would have a regular colonoscopy after 10 years.

There are several surgeons working full-time in Africa who perform the Mainz diversion for selected patients (Michael Breen, Monze Hospital, Zambia, and Sunday Lengmans, Jos Evangel Hospital, Nigeria, personal communications). They are available to deal with any complications and follow-up, and are satisfied that quality of life has been improved at least in the short term. Two encouraging reports of the use of the Mainz diversion have come from Tanzania.[5,6]

We recommend a cautious approach to diversion, giving full weight to the complete physical evaluation as to suitability and a thorough discussion of all the benefits and risks. The patient must never be pressured into an operation – she must make an informed decision and her decision be respected. The operation may be acceptable to the surgeon, but is it acceptable to the patient?

It is my experience that some patients choose to remain as they are after full discussion of the situation. Others may prefer to take a chance of a better quality of life at the price of later morbidity and reduced life expectancy. I have seen several patients who on short-term follow-up are very pleased that they accepted the diversion, but, in my limited experience, the rate of return for follow-up has been disappointing. We badly need more information about the medium-term quality of life and complications so that we can help patients make a responsible choice.

Permanent incontinence is not a happy situation, but perhaps the picture has been coloured by reports of the total rejection that occurs in some communities. In others, we are aware that the incontinent patient is not invariably treated as an outcast – many are cared for by loving families and even their husbands, and they can still live with some dignity.

The Mainz pouch II procedure

The procedure as performed by the surgeons in Mainz[5] involves anastomosis of three limbs of sigmoid colon in an ‘S’ fashion, but most surgeons in Africa have opted for a simpler two-limb anastomosis (Figure 10.3). The Mainz pouch II as performed by Professor Gordon Williams at the Addis Ababa Fistula Hospital is now described and illustrated in Figure 10.4. We recommend that anyone contemplating this procedure should first assist a regular pouch surgeon.

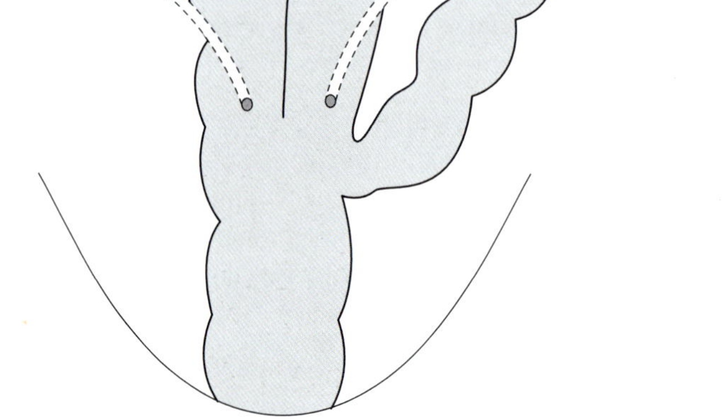

Figure 10.3 In the Mainz pouch II procedure, as practised in Africa, the ureters are usually brought through a small submucosal tunnel low in the back wall of the pouch made from two adjacent loops of sigmoid colon.

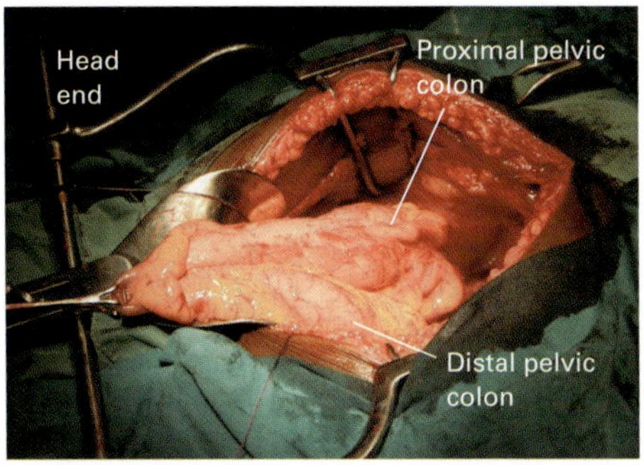

Figure 10.4a The first step is for the abdomen to be opened and for the pelvic colon to be mobilized enough so that it can be lifted out of the abdomen. Using the lower sigmoid the two limbs of the colon are laid side by side and the apex of the pouch is marked with a Babcocks forceps.

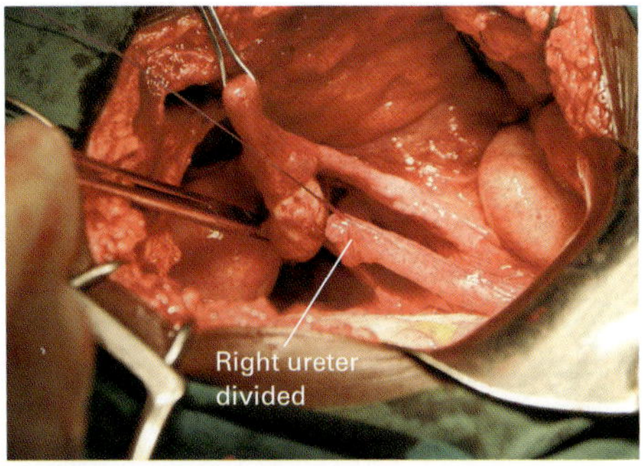

Figure 10.4b Both ureters are mobilized and divided just below the pelvic brim.

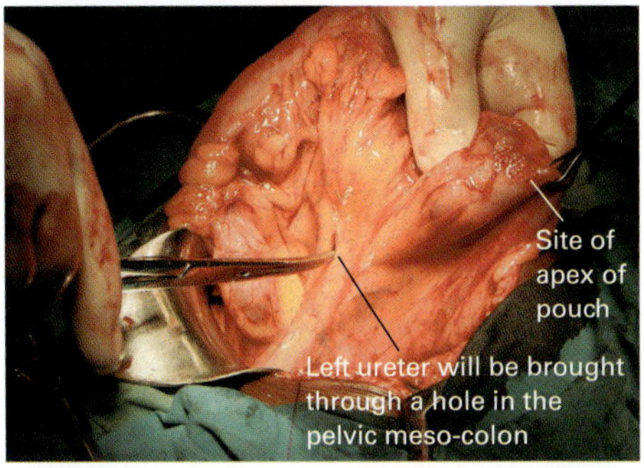

Figure 10.4c The left ureter is drawn though the pelvic meso-colon so that it will reach the pouch without becoming kinked.

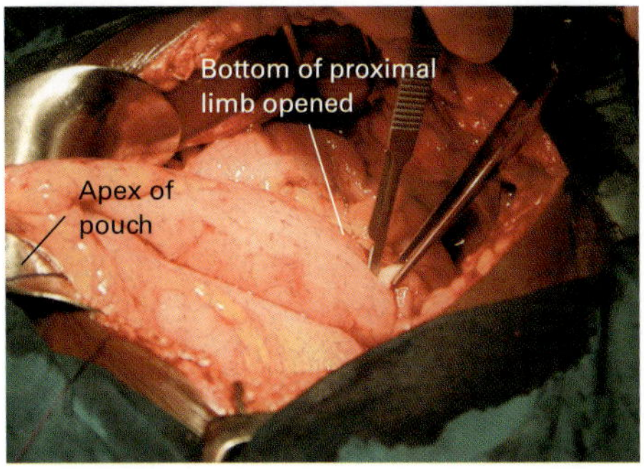

Figure 10.4d The two limbs of the pouch are opened by making a stab incision low in the proximal limb and by then cutting up around the apex and down the second limb.

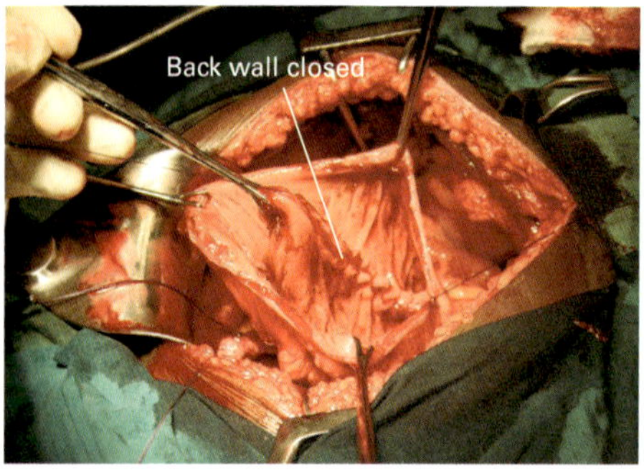

Figure 10.4e After the pouch has been opened, the back wall is closed in one layer.

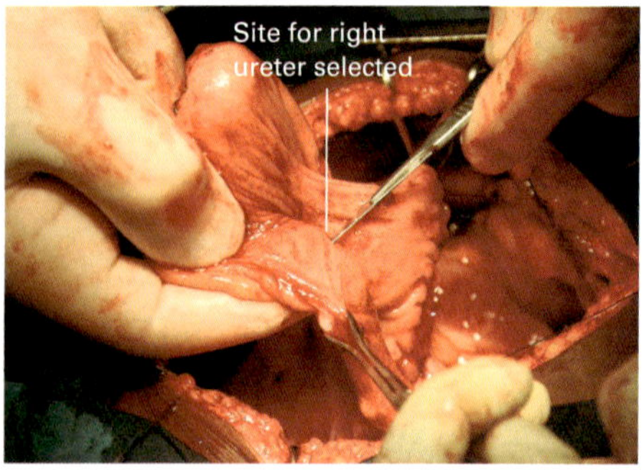

Figure 10.4f A site is then selected in the mid pouch through which to bring the right ureter. A stab incision is made through the mucosa and bowel wall.

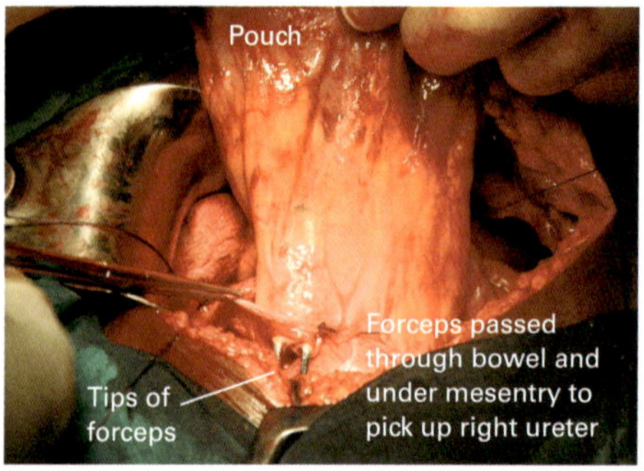

Figure 10.4g Forceps are passed through this incision just under the peritoneum of the meso-colon to reach the right ureter, previously marked with a suture.

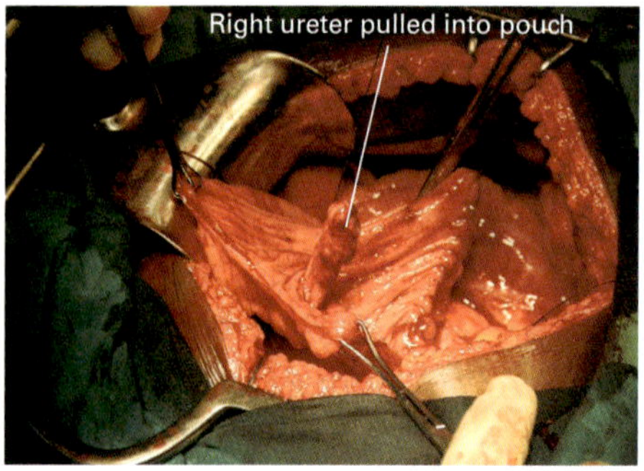

Figure 10.4h The right ureter is grasped by its suture and pulled up into the pouch.

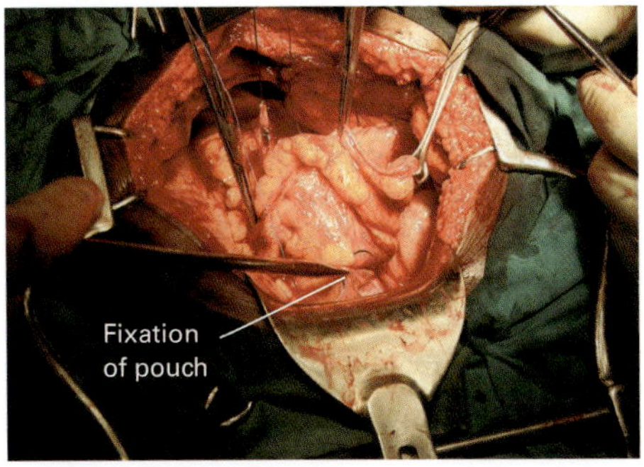

Figure 10.4i After both ureters have been drawn into the pouch it is then a convenient time to insert external sutures to stablize the pouch. Approximately three sutures near the apex of the pouch are inserted into the base of the pelvic meso-colon. Fixing the pouch to the sacral promontory is described in some accounts but seems quite impractical to us.

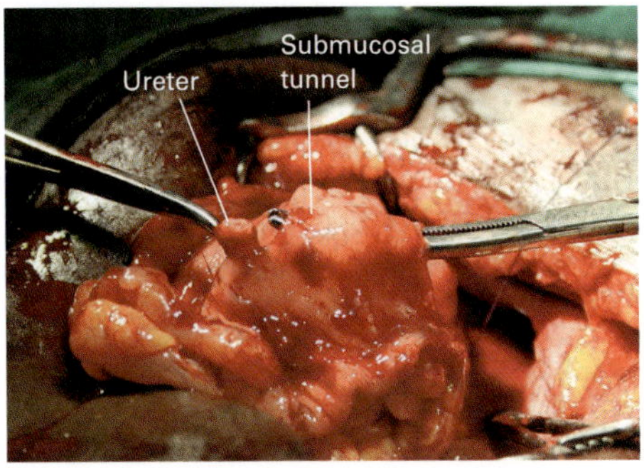

Figure 10.4j A submucosal tunnel is then made to bring the ureter out approximately 2 cm distal in the pouch. A site for the anastomosis is selected and infiltration of the submucosa with saline makes an easier passage for the forceps to pull the ureter through. The first mucosal incision is closed by picking up the adventitia of the ureter at the same time.

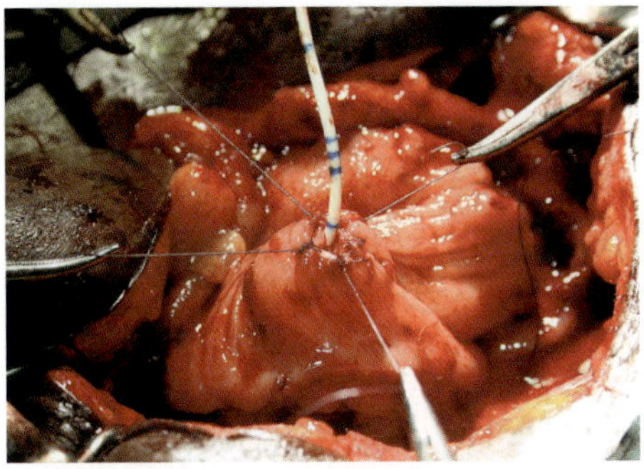

Figure 10.4k After spatulating the ureter, it is accurately anastomosed to the colonic mucosa and sub-mucosa only.

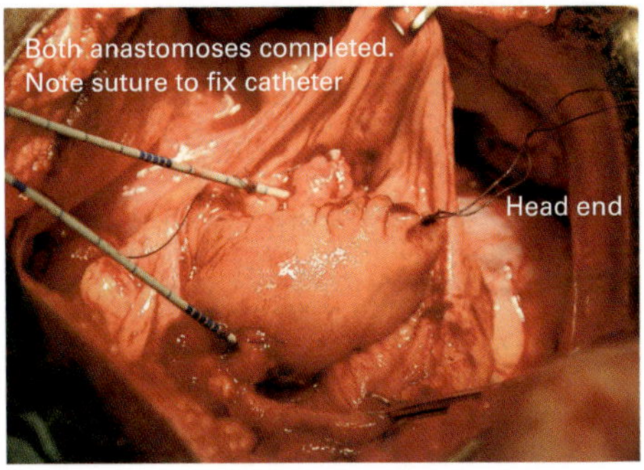

Figure 10.4l The same steps are then repeated with the left ureter. This will also be brought into the pouch under the leaves of the pelvic meso-colon. This ensures that both ureters are entirely under the peritoneum. Both anastomoses are now completed.

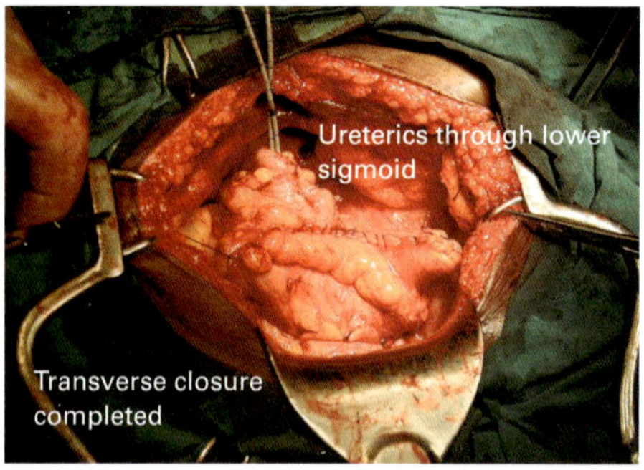

Figure 10.4m The ureteric stents are brought out through the recto-sigmoid about 5 cm below the pouch. A little sero-muscular tunnel is made to bury the catheters for about one cm and they will be brought out through the lower end of the midline incision. The pouch is closed transversely with a continuous suture reinforced by a second layer of interrupted sutures.

The patient must come to theatre with an empty colon. This is achieved by preoperative fluid diet, enemas or, best of all, an osmotic laxative such as sodium picosulphate (Picolax) or mannitol. Single doses of gentamicin 160 mg and metronidazole 500 mg are given intravenously at the start of the operation.

Some surgeons prefer to bring the ureteric catheters out of the anus though a previously inserted rectal tube. We prefer just to use a Foley catheter in the rectum for a few days until the patient is ambulant and can pass urine herself per rectum. Most of the urine drains through the ureteric catheters until they are removed from around the seventh postoperative day.

References

1. Wall LL, Arrowsmith SD, Lassey AT, Danso K. Humanitarian ventures or 'fistula tourism?': the ethical perils of pelvic surgery in the developing world. *Int Urogynecol J Pelvic Floor Dysfunct* 2006; **17**: 559–62.
2. Hodges AM. The Mitrofanoff urinary diversion for complex vesicovaginal fistulae: experience from Uganda. *BJU Int* 1999; **106**: 1227–8.
3. Kees Waaldijk, personal communication.
4. Murray C, Goh J, Fynes M, Carey MP. Urinary and faecal incontinence following delayed primary repair of obstetric fistula. *Br J Obstet Gynaecol* 2002; **109**: 828–32.
5. D'elia G, Pahernik S, Fisch M, Hohenfellner R, Thuroff JW. Mainz Pouch II technique: 10 years' experience. *BJU Int* 2004; **93**: 1037–42.
6. Michael Breen (Monze Hospital, Zambia), personal communication.
7. Sunday Lengmaus (Jos Evangel Hospital, Nigeria), personal communication.
8. Aboud MM. Early outcome of Mainz Pouch 2 urinary diversion. *East Central Afr J Surg* 2001; **6**(2): 15–19.
9. Aboud MM, Eshleman JL, Mteta KA, Mbwambo JS, Oyieko W. An 18-year review of types of continent urinary diversion applicable to the lesser developed regions of Africa. *East Central Afr J Surg* 2000; **5**(1): 17–20.

11 Postoperative Nursing Care of the Fistula Patient

A good operation can be ruined by neglectful aftercare. It is the surgeon's responsibility to ensure that nurses and carers know what is required. In reality, nurses will be in short supply and may be unfamiliar with fistula repair, so postoperative care must be made as simple as possible.

The patient must at all times be:

- draining
- drinking
- dry.

Drainage

Free drainage of urine depends on adequate catheter care. If a catheter blocks, urine may pass alongside it or, *much worse, find a way through the repair.* The scene is then set for failure.

Principles of catheter care

- Nothing must pull on the catheter.
- The catheter must not become blocked or fall out.

The catheter may be secured in the operating theatre with a suture to the mons pubis. This prevents accidental traction on the catheter as the patient is moved from the theatre to the ward and at other times. Strapping to the thigh often comes off, and the catheter may be kinked when the patient turns. Another alternative is to secure the catheter to the abdomen in the midline. Note that there must be slack in the catheter between the urethral orifice and the strapping (Figure 11.1).

Drainage bags or not?

Closed drainage is ideal, but does require vigilant nursing care and good-quality bags (Figure 11.2a). In our experience, the main problem is that the bags may become over-full, especially at night (Figure 11.2b) when nurses are scarce and hampered by frequent power failures. Unless it is certain that staff can look after a drainable bag, we recommend a simple alternative.

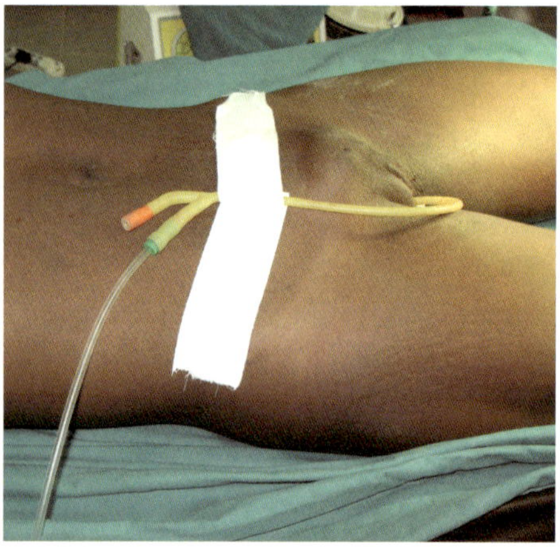

Figure 11.1 There must be some slack in the catheter between the urethral orifice and the strapping.

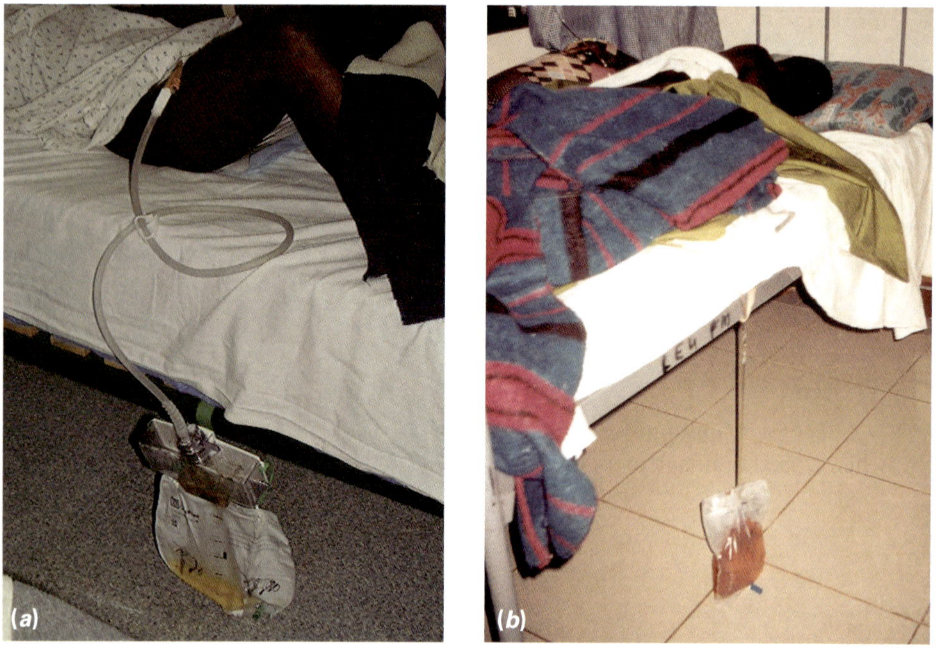

Figure 11.2 (*a*) This high-quality system is ideal, but is expensive and would rarely be available in an African setting. (*b*) This bag has already become full, and if further neglected will over-fill and pull loose from the bed, pulling the catheter out of the patient.

The simplest and safest option is *open catheter drainage*. The catheter is connected to plastic tubing and drains directly into a basin under the bed (Figure 11.3). The patient can move freely in the bed, and nothing will pull on her catheter. It is easy to see that urine is draining by watching the drips, and little can go wrong at night. This is a major consideration when looking after up to 60 patients at once, as on some of our workshops.

Infection does not appear to be a problem if urine output is high.

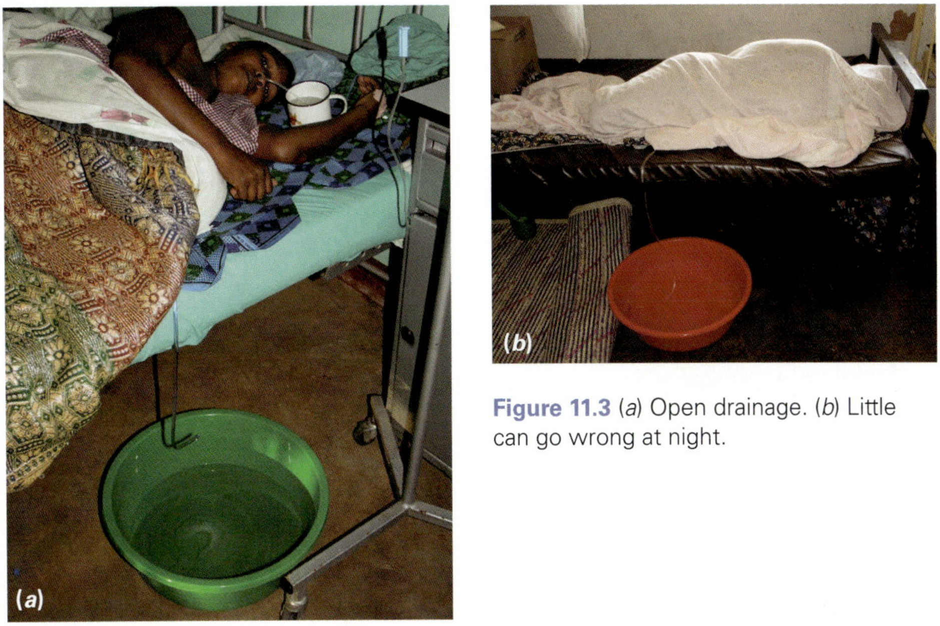

Figure 11.3 (*a*) Open drainage. (*b*) Little can go wrong at night.

Blocked catheter

This is an emergency! The symptoms and signs of a blocked catheter are:

- The patient feels a full bladder.
- She is wet (due to leakage round the catheter or through the repair).
- Urine stops dripping into the basin. This would not be noticed for some time when closed drainage is used.

Action must be taken immediately

- **Examine the catheter** (Figure 11.4). In our experience, a twisted or kinked catheter is the most common cause of cessation of drainage. *Constant vigilance is required by patient and staff.*
- **Examine the patient.** Is the bladder palpable? If so, unblock the catheter at once by gentle saline irrigation with a bladder syringe. Only a maximum of 20 cm^3 are needed. If the bladder is small, there is a danger of overdoing it. If this does not work, change the catheter (Figure 11.5).
- If there is any doubt about drainage, always irrigate the catheter.

Drinking

A high fluid intake is recommended. This should be started before the operation and continued until after removal of the catheter. This means at least 4–5 litres a day.

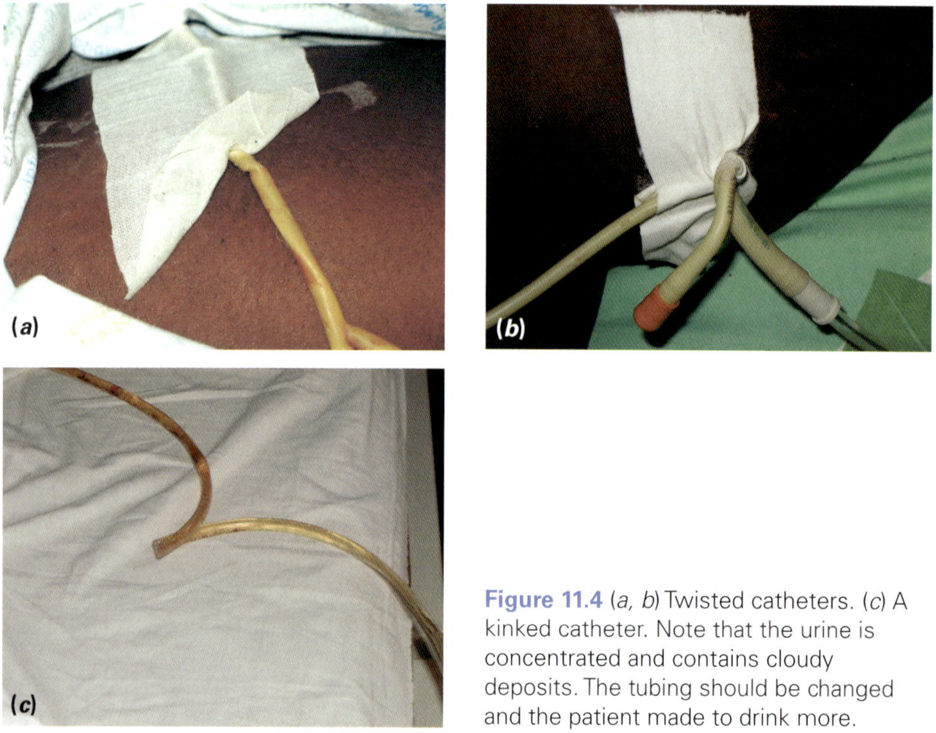

Figure 11.4 (*a, b*) Twisted catheters. (*c*) A kinked catheter. Note that the urine is concentrated and contains cloudy deposits. The tubing should be changed and the patient made to drink more.

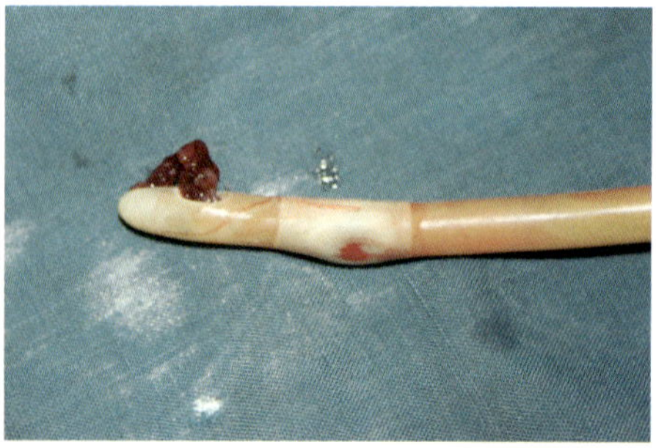

Figure 11.5 This clot caused a blocked catheter on the first postoperative night. Irrigation fluid would go in, but not come out. The clot was acting as a one-way valve. The problem was easily corrected by changing the catheter.

Many patients may be reluctant to drink. They have been accustomed to drinking little to reduce their wetness. They may be afraid that drinking too much will spoil the repair. They should be reassured that this is not so.

Concentrated urine predisposes to urinary infection and to accumulation of debris, which predisposes to blockage.

Drinking can commence as soon as the patient returns from theatre if she had a spinal anaesthetic, and the intravenous line can be discontinued the same evening. The patient should be kept lying flat for 24 hours to reduce the risk of post-spinal headache (Figure 11.6).

There is no need to record urine output except for the immediate postoperative period. With the open drainage method, it is easy to see at a glance whether the

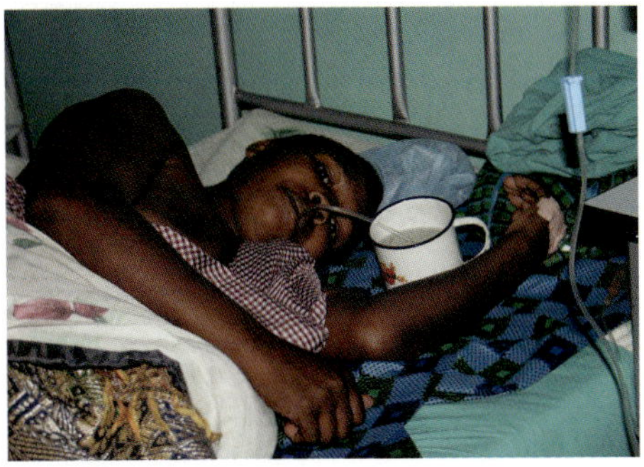

Figure 11.6 The patient is kept lying flat for 24 hours to reduce the risk of post-spinal headache.

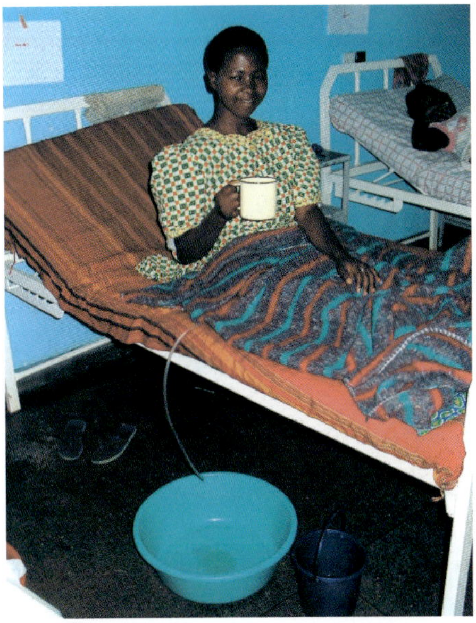

Figure 11.7 The patient must have a plentiful supply of fluids (tea, orange juice or water), and a watch should be kept for urine dripping into the basin.

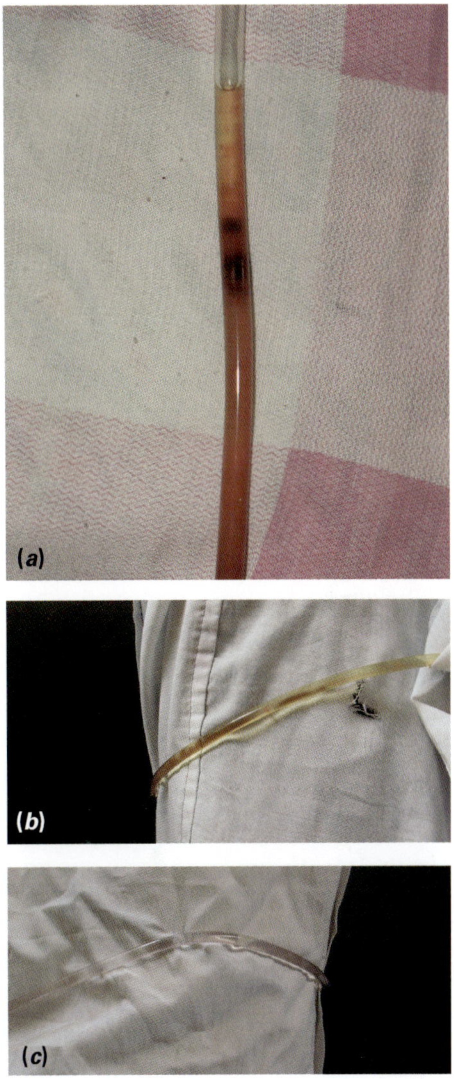

Figure 11.8 (*a*) Dirty, concentrated urine. (*b*) This urine is too concentrated. (*c*) The urine should be like water.

patient is drinking enough. Look for the drips and look at the colour (Figures 11.7 and 11.8).

A word of warning

Occasionally, a patient will take this advice to excess and drink far too much. This can lead to *water intoxication with hyponatraemia*. This presents as confusion and coma, even leading to death. If this is ever suspected, the patient should be treated with 0.9% saline (hypertonic if available) and furosemide to promote diuresis.

Dryness

The patient must be dry. There are several possible causes of wetness:

- The catheter is blocked.
- The repair has failed.
- There is urethral leakage.
- A second fistula has been missed.

Blocked catheter

This is serious, but is easily remedied. It should be uncommon if the patient has a high fluid intake.

Failed repair

This should be very unlikely if the surgeon has selected a simple case and repaired it well. If there is any doubt, a dye test should be performed.

Urethral leakage

As well as draining via the catheter, urine will sometimes leak alongside the catheter, and this may suggest that the urethra has poor function. The typical symptom is that the patient feels wet when standing but not on lying. Careful inspection of the urethra while doing bladder irrigation will identify the problem. Unfortunately, not much can be done.

Sometimes, patients may complain of lower-abdominal cramps accompanied by wetness. This suggests bladder spasms producing a leak around the catheter. Reassure the patient, as these always resolve spontaneously. Hyoscine butylbromide (Buscopan) may help if available.

Missed second fistula

A simple low vesico-vaginal fistula may coexist with an intra-cervical or ureteric fistula (both could be iatrogenic at the time of a caesarean section or a hysterectomy for a ruptured uterus). Note that a dye test at the end of the repair should reveal the cervical fistula (unless it is tiny), but would not show a ureteric leak. A ureteric fistula is easily cured by a second operation to implant the affected ureter into the bladder.

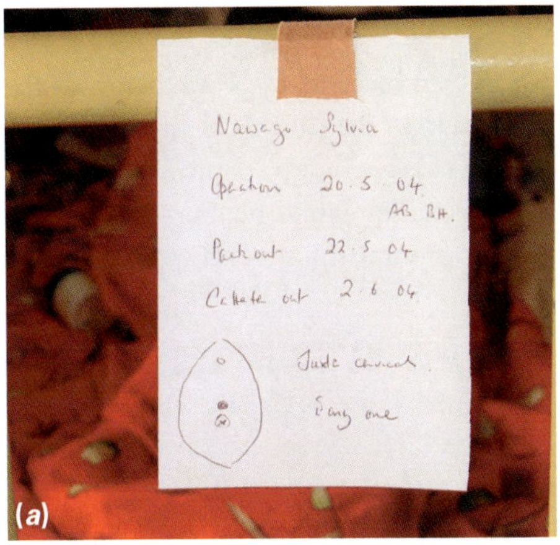

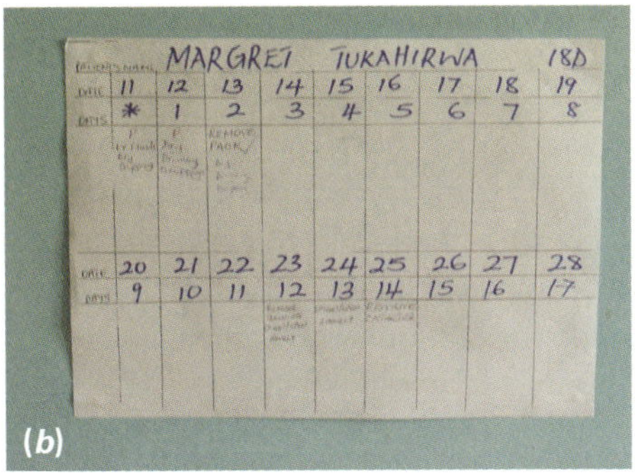

Figure 11.9 A record can be kept at the end of the bed (*a*) or fixed to the wall (*b*).

Record keeping

Keep a simple record of the patient's operation and a postoperative care plan at the foot of the bed or on the wall where it can easily be seen by all (Figure 11.9).

Other aspects of postoperative care

Vaginal packing

Vaginal packing should be removed on day 1 (the day of operation is day 0). There is probably no need to use a pack if the operative field is really dry, but in practice there is often some oozing right to the end of the operation, and most surgeons feel happier to use a pack as a gentle pressure dressing – but it is important to be aware that a vaginal pack can delay the recognition of bleeding deep in the vagina.

Perineal toilet

Twice-daily perineal washing is essential, beginning when the pack is removed on the first postoperative day (Figure 11.10). Particular attention should be given to the catheter as it emerges from the urethra. The patient must perform this washing herself after a few days.

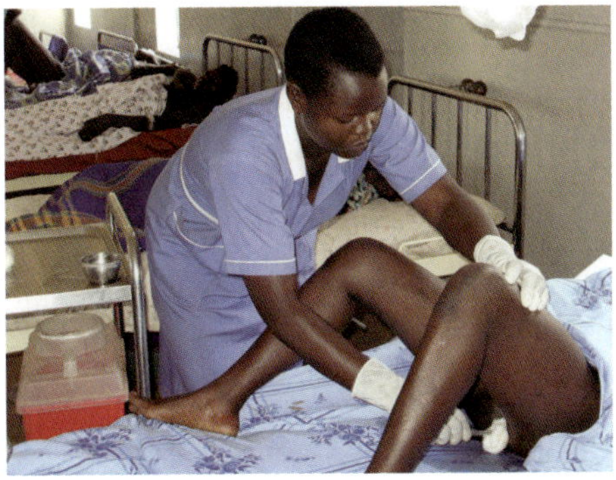

Figure 11.10 Twice-daily perineal care.

Ureteric catheters

Most catheters used to protect the ureters will be removed at the conclusion of the operation. If, however, the repair has been very close to a ureteric orifice or the ureter has been re-implanted into the bladder, the surgeon may require the ureteric catheter to be left in to prevent obstruction to the kidney while healing takes place. It is removed on the surgeon's instructions, usually around the seventh postoperative day, but sometimes after as many as 10 days.

The catheter(s) may be left to drain into a separate bottle (Figure 11.11a), but this hampers early mobility. Two other more convenient methods are illustrated in Figure 11.11(b, c).

Mobilization

The patient is allowed out of bed after removal of the vaginal pack. If she has open drainage, she can use a bucket to collect urine and can carry this around with her (Figure 11.12). This works perfectly well, but it is essential that the patient continues to drink plenty of fluid.

Removal of the catheter

No studies have yet been performed to determine the optimum time for removal of the bladder catheter. From experience, most surgeons leave the catheter in for 14 days after all fistula repairs, but a shorter period may well be sufficient for simple cases. If the catheter is removed earlier, it is essential the patient not be discharged

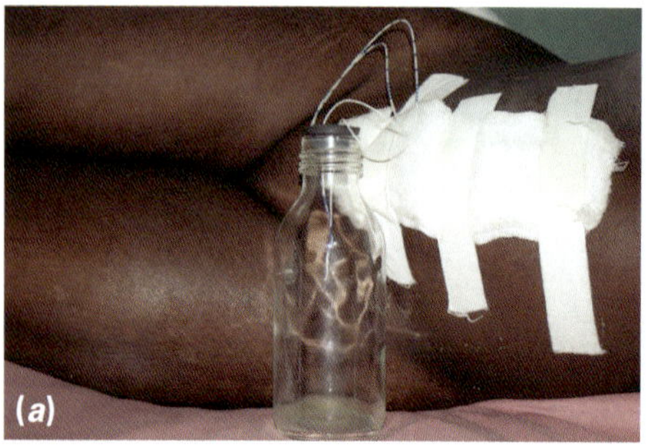

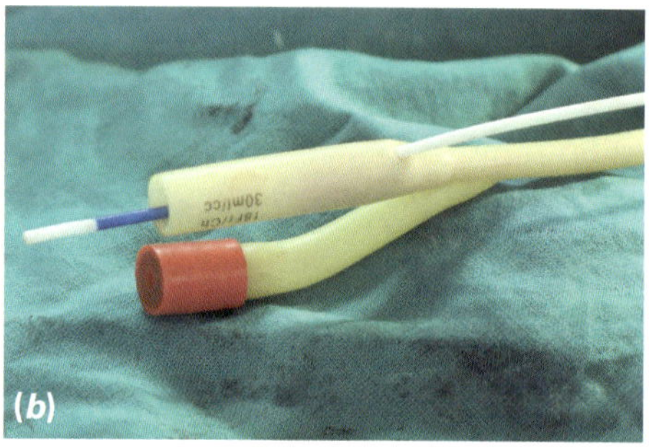

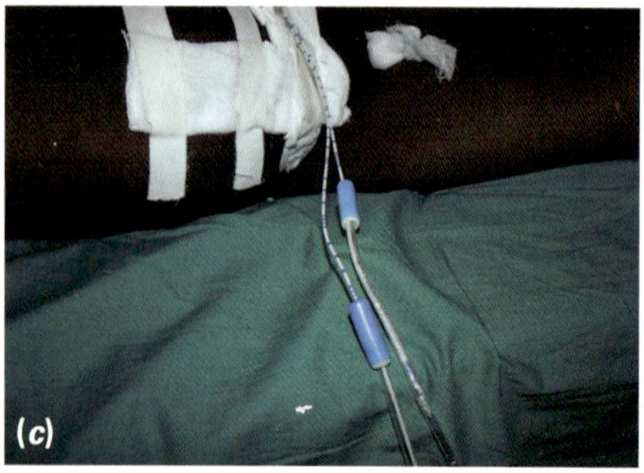

Figure 11.11 (*a*) Traditional ureteric drainage into a bottle. (*b*) The ureteric catheter is placed though a tiny stab incision in the bladder catheter so that they both drain down the same tubing. (*c*) Many drainage bags have a plastic cap on the end. This can be punctured with the point of a towel clip and the ureteric catheter pushed through. It should make a tight fit. This method allows observation of the urine output from each kidney, although this is rarely critical.

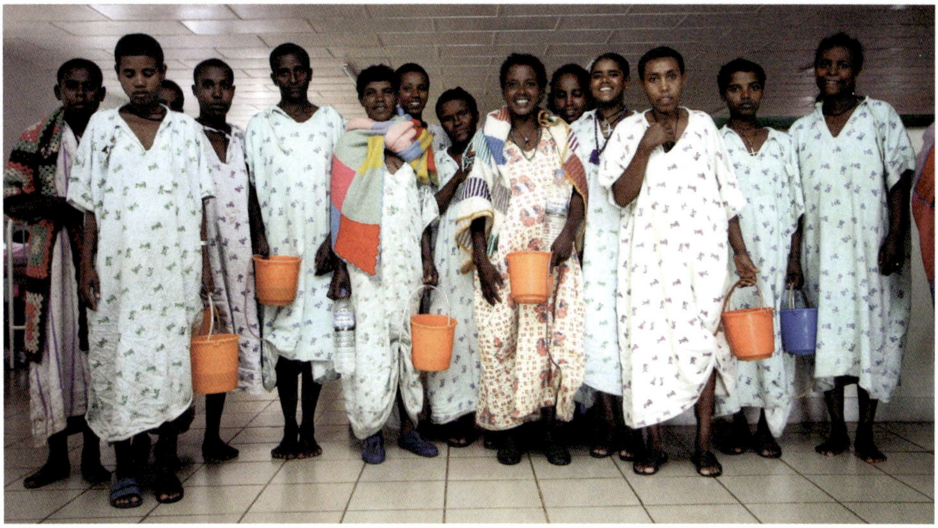

Figure 11.12 Patients up and about with their buckets.

for at least a week, because, if a late breakdown occurs, it can be cured by a further period of bladder drainage,

Some people advocate bladder training, by which they mean intermittent clamping and unclamping for 48 hours before the catheter is due to be removed. With low levels of nursing care, this can easily go wrong if instructions are misunderstood, and we are not convinced that there is any benefit in this regime.

Just before the catheter is due to be removed, it is advisable to perform a dye test in a side room or theatre. This enables the surgeon to determine his or her closure rates and also to note any tendency to urethral leakage. If by chance a small leak from the repair is detected, the bladder must be drained for up to another 2 or even 3 weeks. Small late breakdowns will heal.

It is best to remove the catheter early in the morning and to ask the patient to pass urine frequently. The next day, she can try to hold on longer. If outputs are measured (Figure 11.13), voiding volumes of 25–50 cm^3 are usual on the first day, but rapidly increase to 100–200 cm^3 in most patients.

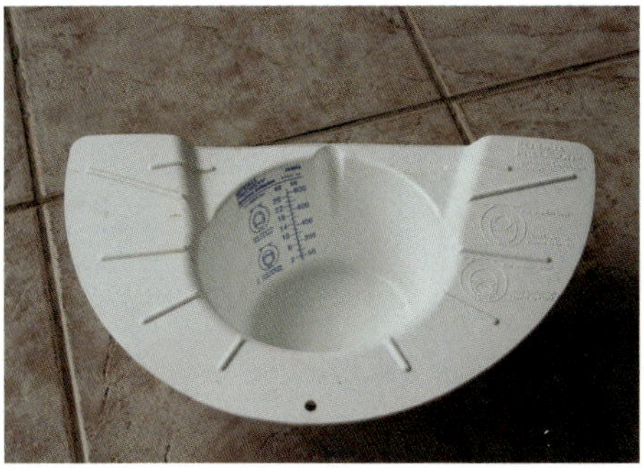

Figure 11.13 A measuring pot that can fit over the toilet.

It is important to be aware that some patients may make frequent attempts to urinate but void little. They are developing retention.

Problems

The patient is wet all the time after removal of the catheter

In this case, the patient has either a totally incompetent urethra or a failed repair; an uncommon cause is retention with overflow incontinence. A dye test is essential to differentiate the first two, and measuring residual urine will detect the latter. A late breakdown must be managed by more catheter drainage, preferably with rest in bed lying prone. If this does not work, the patient must return in 3 months for another attempt at repair. Total incompetence should be treated by teaching pelvic floor exercises (these should ideally be taught before the operation and continued throughout the postoperative period). The prognosis for recovery is poor. The patient should be asked to return in 6 months for further assessment and consideration of a secondary operation for stress incontinence.

The patient can void, but is wet on standing though dry in bed

This suggests a lesser degree of stress incontinence that may improve spontaneously with the help of pelvic floor exercises. We have seen a number of patients who were discharged wet and yet returned for review completely dry.

The patient is dry, but voids frequent small volumes

This strongly suggests retention with overflow, which probably affects about 5% of patients after catheter removal. It is important to enquire if the patient's bladder feels full; if there is any suspicion of retention then the residual urine volume should be measured. If undetected and untreated, the patient will develop overflow incontinence and be predisposed to chronic urine infections. The condition may resolve spontaneously if the bladder is regularly emptied. In dedicated fistula centres, intermittent self-catheterization can be taught, but an easier and sometimes effective option is to discharge the patient with an indwelling catheter. This can be removed after a month, or longer if necessary. It is essential to maintain a high fluid intake to prevent infection.

Failure of repair

A leak requires a dye test unless gentle irrigation demonstrates leakage around the catheter. A leak from the vagina on dye test indicates a failure, but all is not necessarily lost.

Early leak – in the first week

This is bad news, and usually means that the repair has failed. Early leakage should be rare after easy repairs, but is more of a problem in difficult cases. If more urine is draining through the catheter than through the vagina, it is worth keeping the catheter in for as long as this is the case, in the small hope that healing might occur.

Late leak – in the second week or later

Occasionally, even simple repairs develop a leak during the second week. This may be a secondary breakdown due to infection. In these cases, as the fistula margins are not under tension and have good blood supply, there is every chance that the defect will close with prolonged bladder drainage. The catheter should be kept in for up to 3–4 weeks in total, as long as the leak is diminishing.

The later the leak, the better the prognosis

It may help to keep the patient in bed, lying and sleeping face-down (Figure 11.14a). In this position, the hole in the base of the bladder will be uppermost and the catheter tip will be below it, i.e. there is sump drainage (Figure 11.14b, c).

Timing of discharge home

Although, in most cases, the catheter is removed on day 14, *we strongly recommend that the patient does not leave the hospital for a least another week.* We have seen several patients who were said to be dry after catheter removal, but have gone home the next day or two and become wet within days. If they had been able to return immediately and have further catheter drainage, they would probably be healed. They were subsequently found to have very localized breakdown that was easily amenable to a second repair.

Is it advisable to let patients who have had major surgery go home over long distances in crowded taxis, on the back of a bike or by a long walk? It is not surprising that some secondary breakdowns occur. The other advantage of retaining the patient for a week or longer is that one can often see early stress incontinence improving over a matter of days. Also, those with incomplete emptying or urine infections requiring treatment may also be recognized.

All patients must be told to return at once if they become wet after going home, and they should be given money to enable them to do so. They should also be advised to avoid strenuous activity for several months.

The patient should be given a card describing her treatment and giving the operation date to aid later identification and to advise caesarean section should she present pregnant to another hospital.

A cautionary tale

A patient set off on a 200-mile journey home 3 days after removal of a catheter. She claimed to be voiding well. She had a 5-hour ride in a crowded taxi, which did not

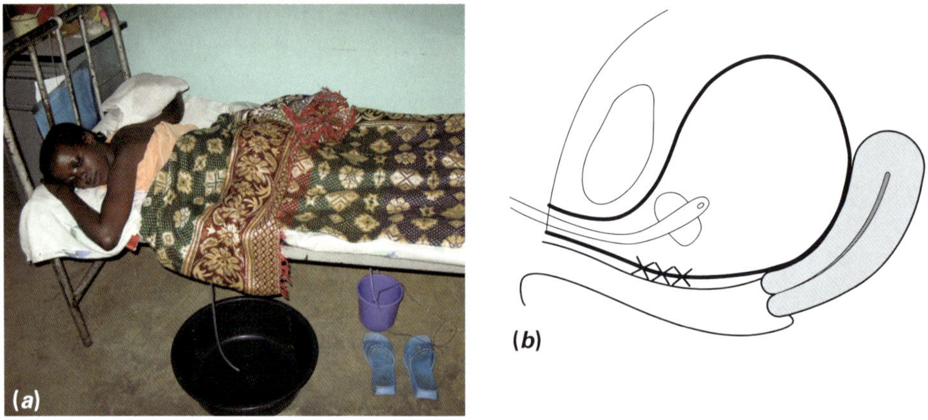

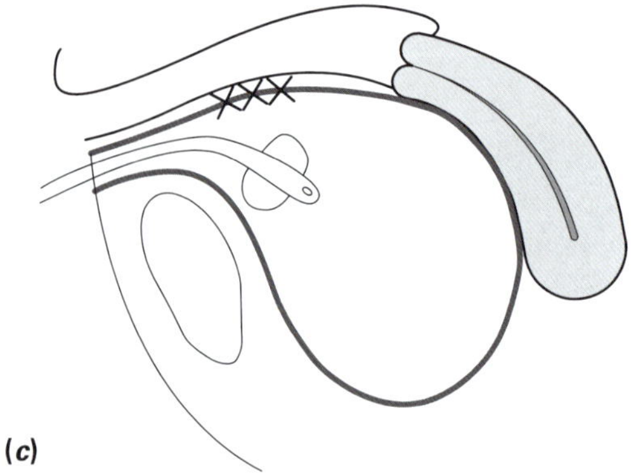

Figure 11.14 (*a*) The patient should be nursed in a prone position if she has a secondary breakdown. (*b*) With the patient on her back, the area of breakdown is in the dependent part of the bladder. (*c*) If the patient lies prone, the defect becomes highest and urine will drain preferentially through the catheter, giving the defect a better chance to heal.

stop on its way. She felt a full bladder, but was too embarrassed to ask the taxi driver to stop. She became wet and, hoping that it was a temporary problem, continued home. Finding herself wet all the time, she was too far to return immediately, and anyway had no money. She later returned. A small, high, very difficult intra-cervical fistula was repaired successfully. If only this patient could have delayed setting off home or returned immediately for further catheter drainage, this situation could have been prevented.

Pre-discharge advice

Counselling

Before discharge, the patient and her family must receive advice so that they understand why the fistula occurred and how it can be prevented in future. Many patients come with traditional beliefs about the cause of the fistula – for example, that it was a punishment for adultery or that someone has cast a spell. These and other false ideas must be gently corrected. Once home, she must become an advocate in her community for prevention.

Abstinence from sexual relationships for at least 3 months

Occasionally, we see patients who went home dry but report a leak developing after a few weeks. Perhaps they were forced into sex.

Caesarean section for all future pregnancies

It is essential to discuss family planning issues, including tubal ligation where relevant. The surest way to maintain a cure is to have no more deliveries! Future pregnancies must be delivered by caesarean section. If the obstructed labour was due to a malpresentation, the patient could possibly deliver vaginally in future, but, as skilled obstetric care is rarely available, it is best to insist on a caesarean section for all subsequent deliveries. From time to time, we do see patients with recurrence of fistulae because they have not been able to get to hospital in time, or because they were given a trial of labour instead of an elective caesarean section.

Return for follow-up consultation

It is so important for surgeons to know their results that patients should be given every encouragement to return. One surgeon forbids resumption of sex until the patient has been seen for follow-up. He gets a high return!

Possible late problems

Urinary infections

With our regime of a single dose of gentamicin 160 mg in theatre and a high urine flow, infected urine is uncommon. A late postoperative infection could be caused by a stricture with retention or even a missed bladder stone. Where limited laboratory facilities exist, inspection of the urine should be enough to make the diagnosis.

Stress incontinence

This frequent and troublesome problem is discussed in Chapter 9.

Stricture

Any patient who had a stricture of the proximal urethra at the time of repair is at risk of postoperative stenosis. Any urinary symptoms require examination of the urethra with dilators. Small Hegar dilators are ideal for this. Small strictures should yield readily to dilatation. Regular dilatation will prevent the stricture from becoming resistant. The patient should be taught to do this herself with a catheter.

Sexual difficulties

In spite of a good repair without any vaginal stenosis, some women are reluctant to resume sexual relations. There may be a number of reasons for this, and sensitive enquiry and examination are required to reassure her. Others with genuine dyspareunia due to vaginal stenosis may be helped by a vaginotomy, especially if the narrowing is localized.

Re-integration

Much has been written about counselling and helping to re-integrate fistula patients into the community. Many patients are very poor and certainly appreciate financial help; however, in practice, if the patient is dry, she will re-integrate and, if she is wet, she may not.

As already mentioned, those patients who are cured must be educated about the cause of their fistula and understand how fistulae should be prevented. They can then become educators for their own community.

12 Assessment of Results

Any surgeon wants to know his or her results, but accurate documentation is beset with a number of difficulties:

- **Inoperable cases.** Specialists vary in their estimates of the percentage that they see as inoperable from the start, ranging from less than 1% to around 5%. Even experienced surgeons can occasionally start a case and find it impossible to finish. Clearly, if these are not included in an analysis then comparison between centres or individuals is not valid.
- **Area of work.** Anyone starting fistula repairs in a new location will have the benefit of virgin territory, with a good proportion of easier cases. As visits or work continue, the percentage of easy cases drops dramatically as re-repairs and cases of stress incontinence dominate the picture. Also, as surgeons become established in their localities, they will be referred more and more difficult cases as surgeons whom they have trained do the easy cases. So the results for the same surgeon may change with time.
- **Incomplete follow-up.** It is ideal practice to perform a dye test before removing a catheter to assess closure rate. If this is not done for all patients, a dye test can be performed just on those who are wet after catheter removal in order to distinguish between breakdown and stress. Some late breakdowns occur after the patient has gone home and some cases of stress cure themselves, so a follow-up appointment is really necessary to be sure of the outcome. However, this is often difficult in an African setting.

Recording results

A key step for any surgeon, whatever his or her experience, is to record results for all new cases and re-repairs separately, and at the same time to diligently record those that are not done because of difficulty or impossibility or that are referred on elsewhere.

We record details of our patients on Excel databases. A balance has to be struck between, on the one hand, collecting every scrap of data just because it might be of future interest and, on the other, missing data that will be useful for prospective analysis. In setting questions, it is important to have 'yes' or 'no' answers or numerical data as in the Goh and Waaldijk classifications. The use of purely descriptive terms for each patient's fistula will not help in the analysis of results. However, there must be a place for describing the operation or other unusual features, as each patient and her fistula are unique.

In assessing results, there are many variables, and one must be clear about definitions:

- **Complete cure**. To be completely cured, the patient must be totally continent and be able to bear children. The only study on fertility after fistula repairs comes from Nigeria, where it was found that only 25% became pregnant again. Reproductive capacity is reduced, the leading causes being amenorrhoea, vaginal stenosis and cervical incompetence.
- **Acceptable cure**. This is to be dry
- **Failure**. This is a breakdown of the repair confirmed by dye test or stress incontinence so bad that the patient feels no improvement on the preoperative state.
- **Stress incontinence**. This occurs in varying degrees and has to be quantified descriptively – and objective assessment is not easy in an African setting. See Chapter 9.

Surgeons working in permanent fistula centres can be much more objective about their results, as they are there to see the early postoperative results themselves, or at least have them accurately assessed by experienced staff.

Throughout Africa, many fistulae are repaired by regular visiting surgeons. They will often have moved on by the time the patient is discharged, and therefore have to rely on later reports from remaining staff, who may for various reasons omit a dye test. This situation obtains to my practice in Uganda and West Africa. A practical method of documentation in this situation is as follows:

- **Cured**. The patient has been seen at least 3 months after her operation and is completely continent.
- **Presumed cured**. The patient was said by the staff to be dry on discharge and has not returned for follow-up.
- **Failure**:
  - The patient became wet in the postoperative period, and breakdown was confirmed by a dye test.
  - The patient was wet on discharge, although it was not known if this was a breakdown or due to stress. A few of the latter cases may improve and not return for follow-up. In our practice, we suspect that the majority who are seriously wet do return. We are then able to decide if they have stress or a broken repair.
- **Stress**. The patient has a negative dye test, but is clearly wet. Further follow-up is needed to decide if this rates as:
  - *Total stress.* The patient feels that she is no better, and she does not void any urine.
  - *Partial stress.* The patient is dry at night on sitting, but becomes wet on walking or standing and does void urine spontaneously.

There will still be a few results that do not comfortably fit into these categories, for example those patients who have strictures requiring dilatation or those with some chronic retention.

We have emphasized that every effort should be made to follow up patients after repair. In addition to enquiry about continence, one should record any changes in menstrual function, sexual function and social integration.

Comparison of results from a part-time versus a full-time fistula surgeon

Given the uncertainties of incomplete follow-up, my best estimate of results as a regular visiting surgeon in 790 consecutive previously untreated cases in Uganda are as follows:

- The fistula is too extensive for any attempt at repair in 2.4% or is irreparable at operation in 1% of cases.
- In 90% of those operated upon, the fistula is closed at the first attempt.
- Of these, there is total stress incontinence in 10% and partial in another 10%.

That is, approximately 70% of new patients go home dry after the first operation.

Andrew Browning's results as a full-time fistula surgeon in Bahr Dar, northern Ethiopia, are considerably better. In 400 new cases, a closure rate of 97.5% was obtained with an 18% urethral incontinence rate at the first operation, i.e. approximately 80% of new patents go home dry after their first operation. About 2% of cases are too bad for any operation.

It is inevitable that a full-time fistula surgeon working in a good environment with a stable team will get better results than an itinerant part-time surgeon such as myself. This is born out by the results recently published by Tom Raassen of his series of 581 previously untreated obstetric fistulae.[1] The setting was the African Medical and Research Foundation (AMREF) Flying Doctor Fistula Project, encompassing 22 different hospitals across Kenya, Tanzania and Uganda. Although the surgeon conducting the repair often departed soon after surgery, the patients were left in the hands of well-trained assistants.

All the patients had a dye test at 14 days, which revealed a successful closure rate of 90.7%; with a further 4-week period of catheter drainage, the closure rate increased to 93.8%. Thus, the dye test had revealed a few unsuspected breakdowns that subsequently healed with further catheter drainage. The stress rate detected at dye test was 8.4%. The symptomatic stress rate may be higher than this.

Another very significant observation was that 16% of patients in the series had had their fistula repaired within 3 months of injury. They did just as well as those who came later for repair.

Mortality rates

Fistula repair is major surgery, and it is not surprising that there will be cases of morbidity and mortality. Mortality of the order of 1 in 500 may be expected. The majority of these deaths will be due to unrelated medical problems. Causes specific to the surgery include anaesthetic mishaps, possible water intoxication and pulmonary embolism. Occasionally, deaths occur for which no clear explanation can be given.

I have so far lost one case from an overwhelming chest infection, and Andrew Browning has also lost one patient from suspected cerebral malaria.

Reference

1. Raassen TJ, Verdaasdonk EGG, Vierhout ME. Prospective results after first time surgery for obstetric fistulas in East African women. *Int Urogynecol J Pelvic Floor Dysfunct* 2008; **19**: 73–9.

13 Problems, Complications and How to Get Out of Trouble

A number of complications may occur during the course of repair, and some of these will be described as learning lessons in how to cope.

Are things not going well?

- Could exposure be improved by larger episiotomies or vaginotomies? Or by more head-down tilt?
- Is the lighting the best that it could be?
- Is the patient slipping down the table? Shoulder rests are essential for a very steep Trendelenberg position, but many operating theatres do not have them. Provided that the patient is placed with her buttocks well over the table with her thighs well flexed, it is possible to obtain 20% of head-down tilt without the patient moving down.
- Are you using an assistant well? An assistant unfamiliar to you should not do anything until asked, and then keep doing it until asked to change. If you have a regular assistant, he or she will be able to anticipate your needs. The most useful skill is to be able to pick up the tip of a needle for the surgeon deep in the vagina (5/8-circle needles make it much easier for surgeons to do this themselves).
- Try to use your assistant as little as possible, and keep the vagina clear of suction devices and instruments. We prefer mostly swabbing ourselves to clear blood and do not use suction as a routine. If flaps are sutured up, there is much less for someone to hold. As Kees Waaldijk has said, 'one person inside the vagina is already a crowd'.

An injured ureter

One of the most embarrassing mishaps is the accidental injury of a ureter at surgery. This has occurred to almost every fistula surgeon – not only beginners. This accident usually happens when mobilizing the bladder in the region of the cervix. Sometimes, the injury is recognized immediately, or it may be noticed at the end of the repair when clear urine is seen escaping.

This accident can be prevented by identifying and catheterizing the ureters at the earliest opportunity during a repair. This is usually done before making any incisions other than vaginotomies, but sometimes it is necessary to begin mobilization before there is any chance of visualizing the orifices. Here, the ureters are at risk, so it is important to avoid straying into the bladder wall and to always keep close to the cervix or stay under the vaginal skin.

It is still possible to cut the ureter with the ureteric catheter in place. If the catheter has a metal stylet, it is advisable to keep it in place during dissection so that it can be felt and so that, if the ureter is cut, it will not be transected. Most catheters do not come with a metal stylet, and on a few occasions surgeons have cut through the ureter and catheter.

Ureteric catheters are not easy to obtain in Africa, and many surgeons who have had some basic training may find themselves without them. The important step is to identify a ureter at risk with a good ureteric probe and, if the ureter needs to be protected, it is possible to use an infant feeding tube (Figure 13.1). Being soft, these tubes are not very easy to insert, and they must be passed through the urethra first. They also slip out easily, and so should be secured by a fine catgut suture in the bladder.

If a ureter is identified as being at risk, it may be possible to protect it without the use of a catheter (Figure 13.2).

How to cope with an injured ureter

There are three approaches:

1. Try to pass the catheter up the real ureteric orifice and 'railroad' it across the gap.
2. Pass a catheter up the cut ureter and fold it into the repair. A cut ureter is more difficult to catheterize in the bladder wall. The lumen may retract. Use the smallest ureteric catheter available.
3. Suture over the cut ureter, finish the repair and implant the ureter into the bladder though a separate abdominal approach.

I have used all three methods with success.

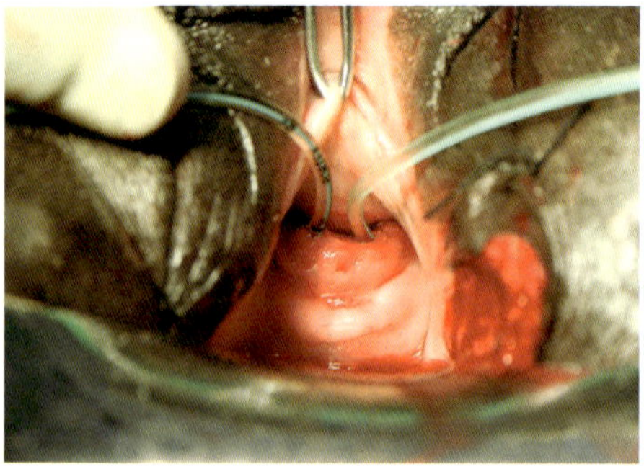

Figure 13.1 Feeding tubes used as ureteric catheters.

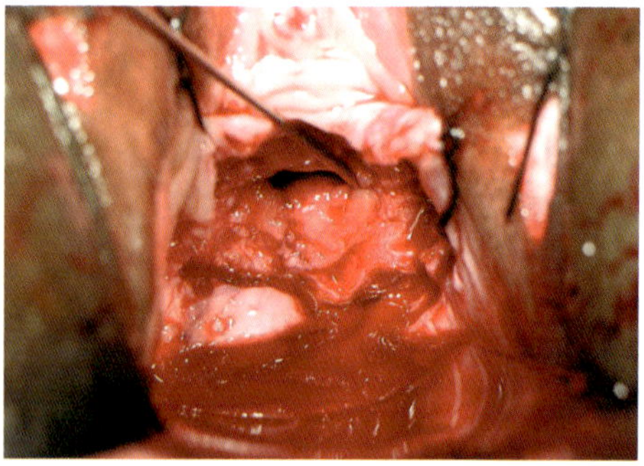

Figure 13.2 A ureter has been identified with a probe. If the distal and proximal corner sutures are placed and tied with the probe in situ, it will not be damaged.

The ureter and the ureteric catheter are cut

I have observed this twice in the hands of very experienced surgeons. The proximal catheter was impossible to extract. The repair was finished and the abdomen opened, the catheter was retrieved and the ureter was implanted into the vault of the bladder.

A trap for the unwary

A double ureter is not that uncommon (Figure 13.3).

An instructive story

A surgeon had completed a difficult repair of a vault fistula without the availability of ureteric catheters. That evening, no urine came through the bladder catheter, but urine was draining down the vagina. Next morning, the patient was taken to theatre. A dye test revealed that the repair was sound. It appeared that one ureter had been ligated and the other damaged in the bladder wall. Ideally, the repair should have been taken down and both ureters identified, but this was impractical. The practical step was to perform a laparotomy and implant both ureters. This was done, with a successful outcome confirmed by 6-month follow-up.

A desperate situation

A patient presented with a recurrent high intra-cervical fistula visible through a split open cervix. The defect extended below the level of the cervix and was judged unsuitable for a trans-vesical repair (Figure 13.4). The ureters were seen squirting on the edge of the ragged defect, but after 45 minutes could not be catheterized. The bladder was mobilized off the cervix remnant and the uterus, and the defect was

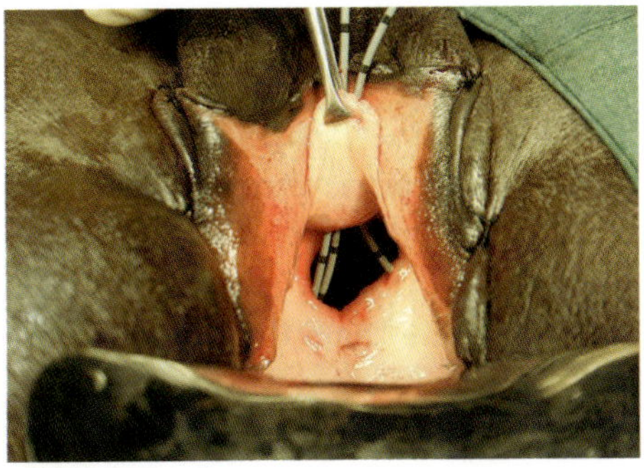

Figure 13.3 A double ureter.

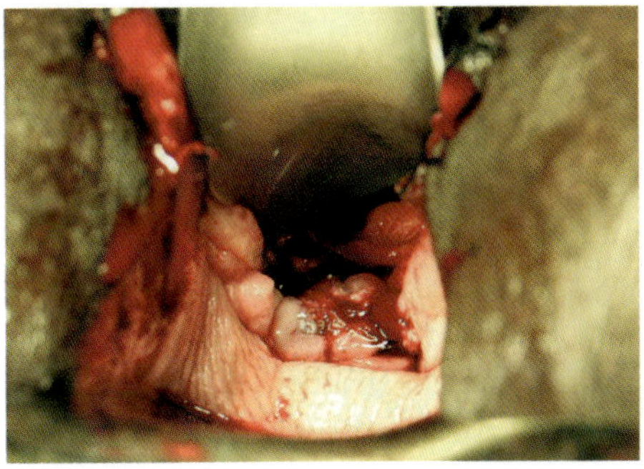

Figure 13.4 View inside the bladder from below. In this case, a deliberate decision was made to close the extensive intra-cervical defect and run the risk of including the ureteric orifices.

closed with a running suture. The ureters were clearly at risk, but there seemed to be no other option. The dye test was negative, but the patient produced no urine on the table. The abdomen was opened, and both dilated ureters were divided and anastomosed to the bladder. The patient had made a complete recovery when she was seen 3 months later.

Miscellaneous mishaps

Intra-vesical bleeding

Bleeding into the bladder should be an exceedingly rare event. We have seen it occur once in the immediate postoperative period. A surgeon had unknowingly entered the plane between bladder mucosa and muscle. It was obvious that heavy bleeding was occurring into the bladder by the appearance of haematuria with clots when the patient returned to the ward. The repair had to be taken down to secure the bleeder in the bladder wall. Although a re-repair was performed, it broke down and was repeated 4 months later.

An injured rectum

At the end of a long day of operating, a surgeon embarked on a difficult repair. In performing vaginotomies to obtain access, he inadvertently opened the rectum. This proved very difficult to repair through all the scar tissue that was present. A colostomy was performed in view of the difficulty. The fistula repair was deferred – it was repaired successfully and the colostomy closed 4 months later.

Lessons

- Do not start a demanding case late in the day.
- Always make vaginotomies just below the 3 and 9 o'clock positions.
- If in doubt, insert a finger into the rectum to act as a guide.

A missed rectal stenosis

I was presented with a patient who had a small circumferential vesico-vaginal (VVF) and a high recto-vaginal (RVF) felt on vaginal examination. The RVF was not palpable on rectal examination. I repaired the VVF and, before starting the RVF repair, I examined the patient per rectum. To my horror, I found that high up there was a complete stricture below the RVF. It would have been impossible to carry out the repair transvaginally. A colostomy was performed, followed by a later resection of the rectal stricture. In spite of considerable faecal contamination, the VVF healed.

Lesson

- It is essential to assess any potential rectal injury fully before embarking on a bladder repair.

Appendix A: Books, Training Material and Suppliers

Books

Moir JC. *The Vesico-Vaginal Fistula*. London: Baillière, Tindall & Cox, 1961 (2nd edn. London: Baillière, Tindall & Cassell, 1967). Out of print, but a limited reprint of the second edition has been produced for the Addis Ababa Fistula Hospital and may be obtained from the hospital at Box 3609, Addis Ababa, Ethiopia, or from Brian Hancock at the address on page 156.

This classic monograph is an excellent introduction to fistula surgery.

Waaldijk K. *Step by Step Surgery of Vesico-Vaginal Fistulas*. Edinburgh: Campion Press, 1994. Available from Teaching Aids at Low Cost (TALC) Box 49, St Albans, Hertfordshire AL1 5TX, UK (info@talcuk.org).

This is valuable reading for any serious fistula surgeon. It is based on Kees Waaldijk's personal experience in Northern Nigeria, which is the largest in the world. It is very detailed and well illustrated, but the beginner might find some parts hard to follow. Dr Waaldijk's experience is constantly evolving and he is embarking on a new series of publications. The first, *Obstetric Fistula Surgery Art and Science: The Basics*, has just been released as a private publication (printed by Printmarkt.eu), obtainable from Dr Waaldijk in the Netherlands (kees.waaldijk@yahoo.com). It contains many gems of wisdom, and his logical classification is clearly explained and illustrated.

Goh J, Krause H. *Female Genital Tract Fistula*. Brisbane: University of Queensland Press, 2004. Available from the Medical Bookshop. University of Queensland. Herston Road, Herston, Queensland 4006, Australia (medicalbookshop@uq.net.au).

This is a comprehensive account of the whole range of obstetric and gynaecological fistulae, but is lacking in specific practical guidance.

Zacharin RF. *Obstetric Fistula*. New York: Springer-Verlag, 1987.

This is an excellent account of the historical aspects of fistula repair, but is of little help to a beginner. It contains a chapter about the early days of the Addis Ababa Fistula Hospital.

Hamlin C (with Little J). *The Hospital by the River*. Sydney: Pan Macmillan Australia, 2001/Oxford: Monarch Books, 2004.

This is a very enjoyable account of Catherine and Reg Hamlin's life and work at the Addis Ababa Fistula Hospital.

Training material

Lewis G, de Bernis L, eds. *Obstetric Fistula: Guiding Principles for Clinical Management and Programme Development.* Geneva: World Health Organization, 2006. Available online at www.who.int/reproductive-health/docs/obstetric_fistula. Hard copy available from World Health Organization, Department of Reproductive Health and Research, Documentation Centre, 1211 Geneva 27, Switzerland (rhrpublications @who.int).

This manual contains chapters on social integration and rehabilitation, nursing care, physiotherapy and operative principles. A summary of the manual is given by de Bernis L. *Int J Gynaecol Obstet* 2007; **99**(suppl 1): S117–21.

Hancock B. *First Steps in Vesico-Vaginal Fistula Repair.* London: Royal Society of Medicine Press, 2005.

This is a practical account for doctors and nurses new to fistula surgery.

Breen M. *Teaching Notes for Obstetric Fistula Repair.* CD, available from Michael Breen, Monze Hospital, PO Box 660029, Monze, Zambia (mbreen@zamnet.zm), or from Brian Hancock at the address below.

This is an amazing resource, consisting of detailed notes of the operative steps for all the major procedures in fistula surgery. In many ways, it is complementary and much more detailed than this present publication. It is based on Michael Breen's extensive experience at Monze Hospital, Zambia.

Teaching Videos (DVD format) from the Addis Ababa Fistula Hospital:

Part 1: Repair of a Simple Vesico-Vaginal Fistula by Catherine Hamlin (40 minutes)

Part 2: Three More Repairs from the Addis Ababa Fistula Hospital (40 minutes).

Obtainable from Brian Hancock, 21 Yealand Rd, Yealand Conyers, Lancashire LA5 9SG, UK (brian@yealand.demon.co.uk).

These videos were made in 1999. Some of the recommendations in the procedures and commentary would now be modified. Part 1 is of particular value as a lasting record of Catherine Hamlin operating and describing so clearly the repairs that she is performing.

Suppliers

Instruments

- Boyd–Stille tonsil scissors (ART No. 101-8420 17 cm)
- Sharp-pointed special Stille–Matarasso scissors (ART No. 101-8458-71)

both from Stille Surgical AB, Sundbybergsvägen 1A, SE-171 73 SOLNA, Sweden (www.stille.se).

- Thorek scissors

from Aesculap (www.surgical-instruments.info).

Clip-on headlight

- Voroscope LED Illumination and Magnification System

from Nuview Ltd, Unit 26, Daniels Industrial Estate, Bath Rd, Stroud, Gloucestershire GL5 3TJ, UK (www.voroscopes.co.uk).

- DC-1 LED Light

from Lemonchase, The Brewery, Bells Yew Green, Tunbridge Wells, Kent TN3 9BD, UK (www.lemonchase.com).

In other countries, similar headlights can be found in resources for dental surgeons.

Needles and sutures

Needles

- *J-shaped fish-hook needles*

from Surgicraft Ltd, 11 The Oaks, Clews Road, Redditch, Worcestershire B98 7ST (www.surgicraft.co.uk or info@surgicraft.co.uk).

Ethicon sutures

- Monocryl 3/0, W3625: 5/8-circle 26 mm round-bodied
- Vicryl 2/0, W9160: 5/8-circle 36 mm round-bodied
- Vicryl 2/0, W9020: Ligapack dispenser reel 2.5 m.

Polysorb sutures

- Polysorb 2/0: Product code UL878 (5/8-circle 27mm needle)

is an excellent suture on a strong, small 5/8-circle needle from Covidien Syneture (www.syneture.com); available in UK from Squadron Medical Ltd (tel: +44(0)1246 470999).

Urethral plugs

These are available from Rochester Medical Corporation, One Rochester Medical Drive, Stewartville, MN 55976, USA (www.rocm.com).

Appendix B: Demographic and Fistula Characteristics

Table B.1 lists some demographic data from our three main hospitals in Uganda (Kitovu, Kamuli and Lira) and the Bahr Dar Fistula Centre in northern Ethiopia. The outstanding difference between the two countries is the frequency of caesarean sections in Uganda – indicating that many people can get to hospital, but arrive too late. In Ethiopia, few people have access to a hospital.

Table B.2 compares primipara with multipara. By all three criteria for a bad fistula – i.e. urethral involvement, circumferential detachment and presence of a recto-vaginal fistula (RVF) – primiparous patients score higher than multiparous patients. This is so for both countries.

Table B.3 compares vaginal delivery with caesarean delivery. Again, by all three criteria, the patients delivering vaginally have significantly more serious injuries than those having their labour relieved by caesarean section. This applies to both countries.

In making comparisons between the two countries, the most striking difference occurred in the primipara (Table B.4), where there was a higher incidence of urethral and circumferential involvement and of recto-vaginal fistula in the Ethiopian patients (p = 0.001). Although the difference in urethral and circumferential involvement could be explained partly by inter-observer variation, a recto-vaginal fistula is always a marker of a severe injury, so it is probable that injuries are more severe in the Ethiopian compared with Ugandan patients, at least among the primipara.

Table B.1 Demographic data

	Uganda	**Ethiopia**
Series	790	606
Not done: considered inoperable (%)	2.4 (19/790)	1.5 (estimate)
For analysis	771	606
Mean age (years)	27	28.8
Mean duration (months)	59	48
Mean time in labour (days)	Not available	3
No. of deliveries per patient	2.9	2.8
Primipara (%)	60	50
Vaginal delivery (%)	34.7	84.5
Caesarean section (%)	65.3	15.5
RVF + VVF (%)	3.3	8.4

Table B.2 Primipara compared with multipara

	Uganda	**Ethiopia**
Primipara		
Number	342	279
Urethral involvement (%)	70	82
(<3.5 cm from external urethral orifice)		
Circumferential (%)	15	41
RVF + VVF (%)	5.3	13.6
Multipara		
Number	417	320
Urethral involvement (%)	51	44
Circumferential (%)	7.7	20
RVF + VVF (%)	1.9	4.3

Table B.3 Vaginal compared with caesarean delivery

	Uganda	**Ethiopia**
Vaginal deliveries		
Number	265	471
Primipara (%)	59.3	50.7
Urethral involvement (%)	77.3	67.8
Circumferential (%)	18.6	32
RVF + VVF (%)	5.2	9.3
Caesarean deliveries		
Number	503	92
Primipara (%)	34	19.5
Urethral involvement (%)	45	30
RVF + VVF (%)	2.4	1

Table B.4 Primipara

	Uganda	**Ethiopia**	***p* value**
Urethral involvement (%)	70.1	81.7	0.009
Circumferential (%)	15.2	40.9	<0.001
RVF + VVF (%)	5.3	13.6	0.001

Acknowledgements

Many people have helped and inspired us to take up fistula surgery, most of all the staff of the Addis Ababa Fistula Hospital.

We would like to dedicate this publication to Dr Catherine Hamlin and her late husband Reg Hamlin, and also to Mamitu Gashe, the patient turned surgeon. Mamitu's skill is legendary, and she assisted and taught us at many of our early repairs, as she has done for so many surgeons who come to learn at the Addis Ababa Fistula Hospital.

We would also like to acknowledge the teaching and example of Dr Kees Waaldijk in Northern Nigeria, who has done so much to train fistula surgeons, contribute to the literature and demonstrate how fistula surgery can be performed with the bare minimum of facilities.

We are extremely grateful for all the stimulating discussions and advice that we have had from so many fistula surgeons. In particular, we acknowledge help from John Kelly, a veteran fistula surgeon who has worked in more African countries than anyone else; from Tom Raassen, the fistula surgeon to the Flying Doctor Service (AMREF), who has dedicated his skill to training so many national surgeons in East

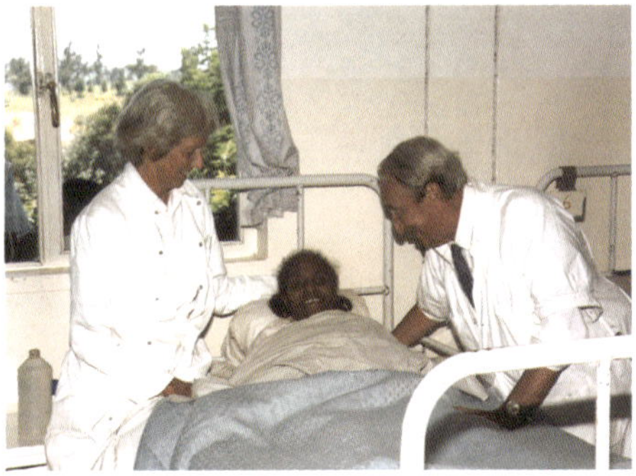

Catherine and Reginald Hamlin in the 1980s.

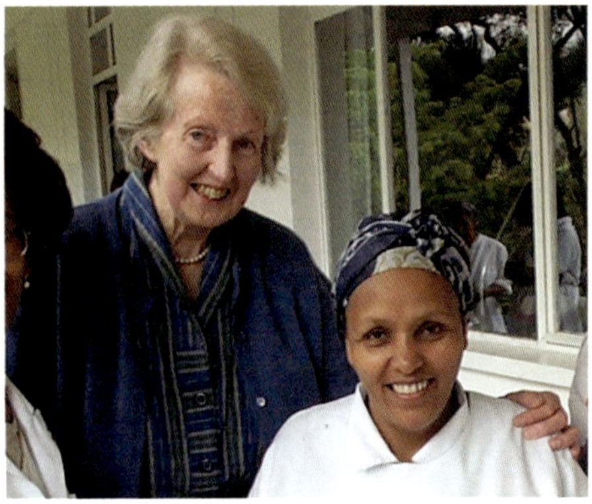

Catherine Hamlin with Mamitu Gashe in 2004.

Africa; from Steven Arrowsmith, VVF coordinator for Mercy Ships; from Judith Goh, a regular contributor to the literature and visiting surgeon to the Addis Ababa Fistula Hospital and Mercy Ships; from Michael Breen from Monze Hospital, Zambia, a great teacher; from Jerry Putman, who got the Aberdeen Fistula Centre in Sierra Leone off to a good start; and from Dr Maura Lynch, who founded the first training centre at Kitovu Hospital, Uganda.

We wish to thank Professor Gordon Williams, Dr Cathrine Reimers, Mike Bishop, Jerry Putman and Harriet Pitt for their valuable comments on the draft manuscript.

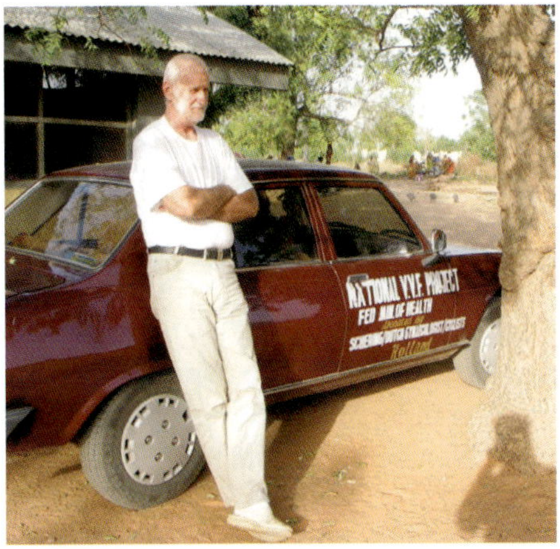

Kees Waaldijk in Katsina, Northern Nigeria.

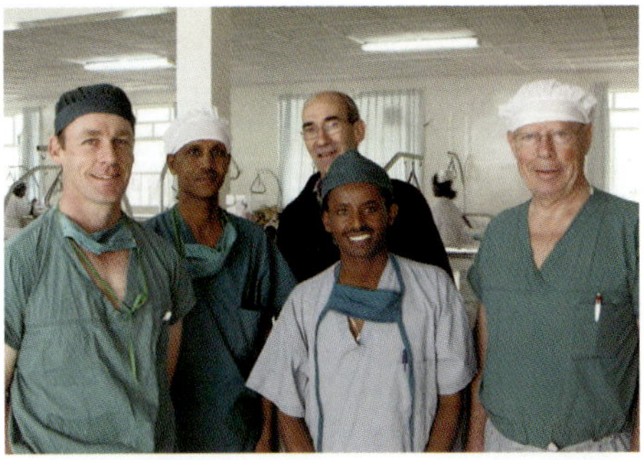

Surgeons at the Addis Ababa Fistula Hospital, August 2008 (left to right: Dr Andrew Browning, Dr Habtemariam, Dr Einar Lande, Dr Hailemariam and Prof Gordon Williams).

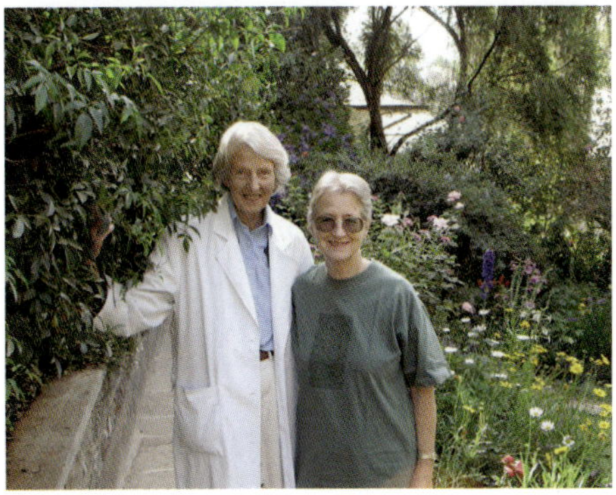

Sister Maura Lynch, seen here with Catherine Hamlin.

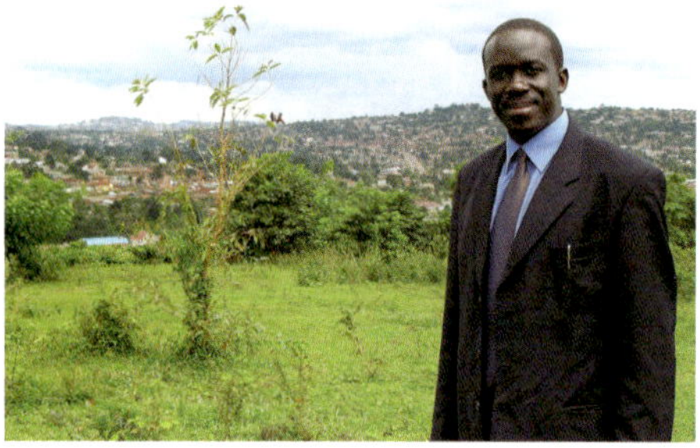

The late Dr William Obote, Senior Lecturer in Surgery, Mulago Hospital and Makerere University, Kampala, Uganda.

We wish to remember our good friend the late Dr William Obote, who took us to Lira Hospital to start fistula surgery in virgin territory and became our mentor in all things Ugandan.

We are most grateful to the following hospitals that have so willingly allowed us to operate and take photographs for use in this book:

- **Uganda**: Kamuli Mission Hospital, Busoga, Eastern Uganda; Kitovu Mission Hospital, Masaka District; Nsambya Mission Hospital, Kampala; Lira Government Hospital, Northern Uganda; Kagando Mission Hospital, Kasese, Western Uganda; Kalongo Mission Hospital, Northern Uganda
- **Nigeria**: Katsina Hospital
- **Ethiopia**: the Addis Ababa Fistula Hospital; the Bahr Dar Fistula Centre
- **Sierra Leone**: Kambia District Government Hospital; Princess Christian Maternity Hospital, Freetown; the Aberdeen Clinic and Fistula Centre
- **Liberia**: Ganta Methodist Hospital, Nimba District
- **Mercy Ships**: in Gambia, Sierra Leone, Benin, Ghana and Liberia (www.mercyships.org).

Index